Higher Sobriety

Jill Stark is an award-winning journalist, author, and mental health advocate, with a career spanning more than two decades in both the UK and Australia. She spent ten years on staff at *The Age* covering health and social affairs as a senior writer and columnist. She now works as a freelance journalist, speechwriter, media consultant, content creator, and public speaker. Her first book, *High Sobriety*, was longlisted for the Walkley Book Award and shortlisted for the Kibble Literary Awards. Her other books, *Happy Never After* and *When You're Not OK*, are mental health memoirs offering hope and connection to anyone doing it tough.

JILL STARK

Higher Sobriety

**MY YEARS
WITHOUT BOOZE**

SCRIBE
Melbourne • London

Scribe Publications
18-20 Edward St, Brunswick, Victoria 3056, Australia
2 John St, Clerkenwell, London, WC1N 2ES, United Kingdom
3754 Pleasant Ave, Suite 100, Minneapolis, Minnesota 55409, USA

Original edition published by Scribe as *High Sobriety* 2013
This edition published 2023

Typeset in Garamond by the publishers

Printed and bound in the UK by CPI Group (UK) Ltd, Croydon CR0 4YY

Scribe is committed to the sustainable use of natural resources and the use
of paper products made responsibly from those resources.

978 1 957363 39 4 (US edition)
978 1 922310 37 8 (Australian edition)
978 1 922586 89 6 (ebook)

scribepublications.com
scribepublications.com.au
scribepublications.co.uk

For Jude, who taught me life's too short to be wasted

THIS BOOK WAS written on the stolen land of the Wurundjeri people of the Kulin Nation, and I pay my deep respects to their Elders, past and present. Aboriginal people are the oldest continuous culture on Earth, and we owe a great debt to their enduring emotional and physical labour in caring for this beautiful country.

I also want to note that this book documents a period in my life when I became an Australian citizen on 26 January 2012 — a date that I knew then as a national celebration called Australia Day. I have since come to understand that 26 January is a day of profound mourning for Indigenous people, marking the beginning of colonisation, invasion, and genocide. If I could have my time again, I would have chosen a different day to become a citizen, but I have decided to leave this section in the updated edition because it's important we learn from our past. I acknowledge First Nations people as the first Australians, and recognise that sovereignty has never been ceded.

Contents

Author's note

THE QUESTION I'VE been asked the most since this book was first released in 2013 is 'What happened next?' The new chapters at the end of this edition attempt to answer that question. So much has changed in a decade — for me and my drinking habits, and for the culture that gave rise to them. While the role of alcohol in our lives was once a topic we might feel apprehensive raising for fear of being branded a killjoy or a wowser, we're now having open and honest conversations about the way we drink. Many people are embracing a different way.

We're witnessing a tectonic shift in drinking patterns, not just in Australia but all over the world. The sober-curious movement is on the march and the non-alcoholic drinks sector is booming, helping to normalise alcohol-free living and making moderation and abstinence more socially acceptable choices. It's an exciting time to be sober.

If you've picked up this book looking to make a change in your life, I hope that it offers some signposts to a road that was once less travelled but is fast becoming a popular path. Cheers to that.

Prologue

THE ROAR IN my skull sounds like waves battering a shore. My head, planted facedown in a sticky pillow, feels as heavy as a waterlogged sandbag. My body is a dance floor for pain. Welcome to 2011, Starkers: a new year, a new start; same old stinking hangover.

Last night was huge. Dawn had broken by the time I staggered home. I remember cursing the light and the chirpy birds. It was, like so many before it, a night that had got away from me. It had been a ridiculously hot Melbourne New Year's Eve: dry and oppressive, with a blasting northerly wind. I felt as if I was trapped inside a fan-forced oven. As I sipped my first drink — a stubby of beer — with friends in their backyard paddling pool, the mercury crept past 40 degrees. It was 6.00 p.m.

As the night wore on, there was champagne with strawberries, more beer, more champagne, and then even more beer. There were sparklers, dancing, and high-pitched phone calls to Scotland, where it was still the last day of the decade before. I vaguely remember a fiercely contested drawing competition with crayons, and, for reasons I can't fathom, sitting atop a stepladder with a miner's lamp strapped to my head.

Later, at another friend's house, we had White Russians in

tumblers, and tequila served in martini glasses. There was raucous laughter, and a Halloween mask, and Lemonheads songs played on a tiny pink guitar. I remember one of my friends vomiting in the kitchen sink, and the group blithely singing over it as if this was neither noteworthy nor unusual. I remember thinking, when's this going to stop? Then having another beer for the road.

I roll over onto my side, releasing a deathbed groan. The alarm clock comes into view, its illuminated digits stabbing my eyes. It's 2.00 p.m. Another groan; this one seems to come from my bones. My guts churn as a tribe of African drummers pounds out a rhythm in my brain, and I pay a grudging respect to a hangover that, having been almost a month in the making, has arrived with some fanfare.

Being conscious hurts. I gag as I think of all the booze I put away in December — one long party interspersed with stolen moments of sleep and tortured days at work.

But covering alcohol is my job. I'm the binge-drinking health reporter. During the week, I write about Australia's booze-soaked culture. At the weekends, I write myself off. For five years I've documented the nation's escalating toll of alcohol abuse as a health reporter for *The Age* and *The Sunday Age*, so I know, more than most, the consequences of risky drinking. I've even won awards for my 'Alcohol Timebomb' series, which highlighted the perilous state of our nation's drinking habits. But it hasn't deterred me. I'm always first on the dance floor and last to leave the party. At the 2010 staff Christmas bash, I won the inaugural Jill Stark Drinking Award. Bestowed upon me for recording the least amount of time between partying and turning up to work, I celebrated the honour with a beer. When colleagues remarked on the irony of my role as health reporter, I told them it was 'gonzo journalism — just immersing myself in the story'. Then I danced into the next morning, breaking my own record by stumbling in to work after four hours' sleep, my title safe for another year.

I stuck the beer-stained certificate on my fridge, ostensibly to show off to friends, but really to serve as a reminder that this was, or should have been, a line in the sand. Yet the festive season leaves little time for self-reflection. There's always another party. I powered on, and on, and on, until the hangover of all hangovers brought me here.

An ungodly noise reverberates around the room. It's impossibly loud. I wrestle with the doona, unearthing my mobile from a pile of clothes. It's my friend and colleague Nat. I can't talk to her. The inside of my head is a graveyard for brain cells. Those that survived last night are clinging to life, resting on the backs of their fallen comrades, too weak to help me form words. I turn the phone to silent, waiting for the message-bank alert to vibrate.

'Hi darl, happy new year!' Nat trills in her singsong voice. 'So sorry to bother you on your day off, but I really need your help. Brendan Fevola's been arrested for being drunk, and I have to do the story. I need to find some alcohol experts to talk about whether he should be in rehab, is his career over, where to next, that sort of thing. Was hoping you'd be able to put me on to some of your contacts. Anyway, hope you had a good night. If you can call me back, that would be great.'

It's an hour before I recover the motor skills to send Nat the contacts. Scrolling through my phone, I find the mobile numbers of Australia's leading authorities on alcohol abuse. The chief executive of the Australian Drug Foundation, the chairman of the National Health and Medical Research Council's working committee on alcohol, the head of the prime minister's National Preventative Health Taskforce: these are men who trust and respect me, men who will draw on their decades of expertise to speak eloquently on the best road to rehabilitation for a troubled star footballer who has had one big night too many. Fev will be in good hands.

But what about me? As I lie here, enveloped by a sense of shame and the stench of stale pale ale, the only thing louder than the thumping pain in my head is a noise I have tried to ignore for months: the tick, tick, tick of my own alcohol timebomb.

I'VE BEEN A binge drinker since I was a teenager. Growing up in Scotland, a place where whisky outsells milk, and teetotalism is a crime punishable by death, devotion to drinking is as much a part of my national identity as tartan, bagpipes, and arctic weather conditions.

I had my first drink at 13 — a can of lager that my best friend, Fiona, and I stole from my parents' drinks cabinet. We laced it with sugar in a failed attempt to make it taste less revolting, and drank it through a straw because we'd heard this would get us pissed faster. It would take many years before I warmed to the taste of alcohol, but I immediately fell in love with being drunk. It felt freeing, exhilarating, and endlessly fun and hilarious. It opened up a world where life's sharp corners were blunted, and worries melted like chocolate on a sunny dashboard. I couldn't believe it was legal.

Since then, I've rarely questioned my big weekends. Getting drunk is the social norm, and as much a part of life as eating and sleeping. When I moved to Australia in my mid-twenties, I was delighted to discover that my adopted country had a similar affection for alcohol, and was even more excited to learn that not only could you drink beer at the football, but also that every year on the first Tuesday in November you got a day off to get pissed and watch a horse race. This was my kind of place.

Many times I've vowed 'never again', as what begins as a few quiet drinks invariably turns into a lost weekend. Then, when the hangover fades to a dull memory, I do it again. Alcohol accompanies almost every aspect of my social life: parties, gigs, dinners, birthdays, holidays, book club, work functions. Even my dance class is held in a pub. Drinking socially has become an act as automatic as breathing.

But something has changed in recent months. My 35th birthday looms, I have a grown-up job and a ridiculous mortgage, and my knees now make a cracking noise every time I stand up. I can no longer afford to drink as though I'm a teenager. The hangovers are hitting harder and lasting longer. A big night out can leave me feeling flat for days. It's not until now, my New Year's Day nightmare, that I realise just how big a price I'm paying.

After texting Nat the numbers, I doze off for an hour or so, not ready to deal with all that a new year represents. A bad dream wakes me up with a jolt, and I lie there motionless, staring at the ceiling — too tired to move, too jumpy to sleep.

Then I feel it: the slow creep of panic. It starts, as it always does, with a tingling sensation around my heart, rising feverishly until it feels as if my heart might shatter or burst right out of my chest. Pins and needles run through my fingers. My feet turn to slabs of stone. My breathing is so laboured that I have to remind myself to inhale and exhale.

I first began to suffer panic attacks as a teenager. Over time, I learned to control them to the point where they rarely bothered me, but recently they've crept back. Hangovers are often the trigger.

On this first day of 2011, the panic returns with a fury I'd forgotten. It comes in waves, racking my body and rising up to my brain with a rush of blood that makes my head sway. My heart, beating as fast as a champion racehorse, is so loud it's all I can hear. I feel like I might pass out. Or die. Each surge brings more thoughts that trigger more waves of panic. What's happening to me? *Surge.* I haven't felt like this for years. *Wave.* Maybe I should eat something. *Surge.*

Even the idea of buttering toast is more than I can handle. But I'm light-headed and hungry. I throw on jeans and a T-shirt, and jump in the car to go to McDonald's.

Big mistake.

I make it out of my garage, and I'm at the traffic lights when it comes: a wave of panic so powerful that it takes all my strength not to run screaming from the car. Traffic is behind me, pedestrians are on the crossing, and I'm facing a red light. To my right, a metallic-blue Mitsubishi Lancer with tinted windows is pulsating to music that could best be described as angry noise. As I turn the radio on to drown it out, the sight of my trembling hand triggers another wave of panic. The DJ bursts forth from the speakers, babbling about new year's resolutions and hangover cures. I can't cope. I mash the buttons with the palm of my hand like an elephant trying to master a typewriter. Breathe. Remember to breathe.

The lights turn green and I turn left. I've only travelled a few metres when another wave threatens to run me off the road. I pull over into a side street, head between my legs, willing myself to keep it together. 'You can do this, Starkers,' I incant, breathing slow and hard, in through my nose and out through my mouth, as I first learned when I was a petrified 16-year-old — half a lifetime ago.

I compose myself enough to continue the short drive. The panic seems to subside marginally when I'm moving; stationary, everything turns to custard. At the drive-through, I pray for a swift getaway. It's not my day. The man in the Ford Falcon in front is ordering enough for a footy team. Fuck him and his four Quarter Pounders, six Big Macs, and three Happy Meals! Resting my forehead on the steering wheel, I manage a wry smile, wondering if Fev's morning-after is filled with similar dramas. Anxiety doesn't like this; it kicks me up the rear end with another surge of panic. Cars are backing up behind me — more New Year's Eve casualties in search of just the right combination of fat, salt, and sugar to ease their pain.

Finally, the hungriest man in Melbourne finishes his order. When it's my turn, I bristle at the sound of my voice. It's distant and disembodied. The girl who takes my money is apprehensive. I wasn't game enough to look in the mirror before I left the house, but I suspect it isn't pretty.

Back home, I curl up on the couch, munching my foul-smelling meal like a rat gnawing on a bone. Still the panic comes, but the waves begin to lap more gently as exhaustion kicks in. I crawl back into bed around 9.00 p.m., the first day of a new year a complete write-off. I'm broken. No party is worth this much pain.

Before

FOR MONTHS, I'VE been thinking about taking a break from alcohol. When I say 'thinking about it', I mean toying with the idea for a few minutes in the depths of a raging hangover, before dismissing it as an exercise in planned insanity. But the thought hasn't gone away. Each new morning-after brings another set of what-ifs. What if the Monday-morning condition I've come to think of as 'wee bit fuzzy brain' is something more sinister? What if those moments where I can't articulate the words that seem to be bogged in a quagmire somewhere between my mind and my mouth are a warning that shit-faced shenanigans can't be sustained as a lifetime sport? Is my body about to express its protest at two decades' worth of abuse by rebelling against me in a way that can't be cleansed with a Sunday-afternoon sleep-in?

My hangovers are no longer carefree retreats under a doona with the weekend papers. They've become fraught with anxiety, pain, and a hint of guilt — the root of which I can't quite place. It pisses me off. All I want to do is wallow in my morning-after, park my arse on the couch, and eat a packet of Tim Tams in front of *The Biggest Loser*. But the thoughts won't let me rest; they niggle and taunt. The loudest and most persistent reminds me with annoying frequency that my life can be summed up in two words: working and drinking. When I speak to my parents in Scotland and they ask what's new, these are the things that most readily come to mind. I don't drink alone, and rarely at home. But socially, I can't remember the last time I turned down a beer or a glass of wine.

I'm not unique; I'm surrounded by people who drink in exactly the same way. I grew up in a country devoted to boozing, and I moved to a nation similarly enamoured with it. Just like Scotland, Australia's default bonding-ritual is drinking. We use it to celebrate, commiserate, and commemorate. Getting plastered is a rite of passage for teenagers, and it's also the accepted and expected way to mark any major celebration. Drinking is how we farewell the dead and welcome the newly arrived; we drink at the footy, we drink with workmates, we drink on public holidays and on weekends. Booze is the nation's social lifeblood.

Against this backdrop, quitting seems impossible. I cannot and do not want to imagine a life without alcohol. If I have to pick one word to describe what it might be like, it would simply be 'boring'. The drawbacks of not drinking far outweigh the unknown, and in no way guaranteed, advantages of abstinence; if I ditch alcohol I'll be casting myself adrift into the social wilderness, a place from which there might be no return. Most of the non-drinkers I know are either pregnant or pensioners. As I'm neither, I've opted to keep drinking until whichever of those fates befalls me first.

But still, the niggling thoughts prevail. What would it take for me to stop drinking? Why does the idea of doing so scare the bejesus out of me?

Those thoughts were first planted in my mind almost a year ago, after meeting Chris Raine. This party-hardened young advertising professional from Queensland's Sunshine Coast gave up drinking for a year — partly as a social experiment and partly because his friends told him he couldn't — and documented the experience on a blog,

Hello Sunday Morning. His insights into his relationship with alcohol inspired some of his friends to follow suit. Soon the site became home to a community of those taking a break from drinking. When I looked at it, I was struck by the potential of what he'd started. Here was a network of young people all enjoying life and achieving their goals, simply by cutting out booze for three, six, or 12 months, and blogging about their experiences. This public commitment was the key to the movement's success, helping to keep people accountable, and therefore boosting their chances of making the distance. Posting links to their blogs on Twitter and Facebook had a ripple effect, encouraging others in each writer's social network to take up the challenge.

There were fewer than 50 bloggers when I first visited the *Hello Sunday Morning* website, but the unflinching honesty in their posts was powerful. These were young people, largely in their twenties, drowning in a culture that implored them to drink at every juncture. What I found disarming was how dissatisfied they were with the culture they'd inherited — but they knew no other way. They drank to fit in; they drank for confidence; they drank to deal with difficult emotions. They drank because it would be social suicide not to. I realised that in all of the alcohol stories I'd written, I hadn't come close to capturing what Chris had harnessed. He'd figured out what politicians, journalists, and health experts had failed to: why young people from Cairns to Castlemaine were regularly drinking themselves into oblivion.

Public-health experts have been telling me for years that, if we are to have a chance of reducing the enormous medical, social, and economic burden of alcohol misuse, we first have to change Australia's entrenched binge-drinking culture. We can no longer debate that there is a problem. Every week, four Australians under the age of 25 die, and 60 teenagers are hospitalised, due to alcohol-related injuries. Between 1997 and 2007, the number of young people treated for alcohol-related brain damage grew five-fold.

But working out how to reach these drinkers has proved a tricky proposition. Governments have thrown money at campaigns demonising booze, and warning young people that drinking will see them arrested, maimed, raped, or killed. The testimonies of Chris and his fellow bloggers reveal that this approach has left young people feeling patronised and alienated. It's given them no incentive to change their drinking habits, and may well have encouraged them to veer in the opposite direction in protest. While I'd be flattering myself to think I'm in the youth demographic these campaigns have been trying to reach, I've been equally turned off by messages which imply that drinking is inherently dangerous and unpleasant, when my own experiences tell quite a different story. I could see how what Chris had come up with might well be the road map to reach a disillusioned generation.

When I first interviewed him over the phone, where he spoke to me from his Caloundra home, I was astonished by his level of insight into the complex connections that Aussies have with alcohol. His ability to articulate his own motivations for drinking was even more impressive, especially for someone who was just 23. I remember wondering where I'd be now if I'd had that degree of clarity about my own relationship with alcohol at his age.

In early 2010, Chris and I met in person. Relentlessly upbeat and energetic, he had a passion for his work that coursed through him so violently he was practically luminous. Here was a man on a mission — to change our drinking culture and to unlock what he believed to be Australia's greatest untapped resource: Sunday mornings. And his pitch was convincing. 'We live in a country where we're hung-over for a seventh of our lives. If you binge drink for two nights a week between the ages of 18 and 28, you'll have drunk for 10,000 hours. We're creating a culture of drinking experts,' he told me. 'The cost of that expertise is 3000 people a year dying from alcohol misuse. That's 57 Australians every single week.' Chris reckoned that three months off the booze was the minimum time it took to fundamentally shift a person's relationship with alcohol.

I admired what he was trying to achieve, but I was also a little suspicious. Was *Hello Sunday Morning* a modern-day temperance movement? A slick front for God-bothering puritans?

But there was something about him. On some level, even then, I knew that meeting Chris was a game-changer. I quizzed him on his year without booze. Didn't he get bored? How could he enjoy parties without a few beers? A whole year? Seriously? I accused him of being a lentil-loving tree hugger on a mission to change the world one booze-ravaged soul at a time. He would offer only a chuckle and the suggestion that I should try it for myself if I wanted to find out how it worked.

Gradually, as my doubts about Chris dissipated, I could see what I really doubted — my ability to forgo alcohol for what seemed like a preposterously long period. I'd given up booze before: prior to meeting Chris, I'd just finished Febfast, in which participants give up drinking during February to raise money for young people with drug and alcohol problems. But it was a white-knuckle ride. I put life on hold, waiting out my booze ban like a footballer pacing the sidelines, desperate to get back in the game. I struggled to imagine how, if I removed alcohol for an even longer period, life could be anything short of two-dimensional. Don't the best nights out usually happen after a skinful? Hedonism rarely springs from soda water. I had more faith in the transcending power of beer than I did in myself.

The hangovers continued after meeting Chris, and the what-ifs lobbed into my mind with increasing regularity. I did my best to ignore them. That's not easy when you spend your working life writing about the health consequences of a society sickening itself on a noxious diet of booze, fags, and fast food — the public-health world's axis of evil. Health reporting can induce the sort of hypochondria that would make Woody Allen proud. But some health messages I chose to ignore; I had only stubbed my last cigarette out a couple of years before. It had taken several weeks of waking up in the middle of the night with coughing fits that made my abdominal muscles ache before I finally called it a day. Sometimes the only way you can change is when the future slaps you in the face so hard it leaves a handprint on your cheek.

But smoking's not like drinking. These days, it's almost more socially acceptable to marry your cousin than to light up in a public place. With alcohol, the opposite is true. If you want to be a social pariah, try refusing a drink in an Australian pub at six o'clock on a Friday evening. I've had no doomsday warning with booze — and even if there had been one, I've mastered the art of selective hearing. I paid scant attention to the implications of a story I wrote about research which warned that as little as eight drinks a week could shrink the size of your brain. But a study that found regular drinkers have above-average happiness and wellbeing scores, while non-drinkers are the most miserable, was digested in great detail and posted on my Facebook page.

For me, being drunk was not a fast track to ill health and calamity. I was binge drinking before the phrase was even invented, and so were most of my friends. We're all still alive and healthy. We haven't been in car accidents, been assaulted, or assaulted someone else. We haven't woken up in hospitals, contracted communicable diseases, lost jobs, committed crimes (barring crimes against music in karaoke bars), ruined relationships, or gambled away our life savings on the pokies as a result of our drinking. For the most part, being drunk is fun for us. It brings texture to our lives, and leads to new friendships, dancing, romance, sex, belly laughs, and bonding. The stories I write for my newspaper about alcohol-induced carnage simply don't resonate with my own experiences. The soaring rates of alcohol-related injuries and liver disease, the brain-damaged women, and their kids being born with foetal alcohol syndrome — I might as well be writing about life on another planet.

Reporting on alcohol might have become the defining issue of my journalistic career, but I merely convey facts. I can't comfortably be likened to the politician who preaches family values while secretly committing acts of depravity with leather-clad call girls. In my mind, I'm no more obliged to drink responsibly than the transport reporter is obliged to ride his bike to work to ease Melbourne's traffic congestion.

Still, I have to admit that my two worlds sometimes collide. A year or so into my coverage of Australia's binge-drinking epidemic, I had a boozy Saturday-night dinner party with some girlfriends and got to bed around 2.30 a.m., waking up, with a scratchy throat and a sore head, around six hours later to go to work. I was hoping for a quiet Sunday shift, with something light and inoffensive that would glide its way inconspicuously onto page 12 — perhaps a colour piece on a charity fun-run, or a discussion on the best treatments for baldness. Instead, I learned that overnight the federal government had announced that taxes on pre-mixed spirits, colloquially known as 'alcopops', would be raised by 70 per cent, effective immediately. As I was the resident expert on all things binge drinking, and alcopops had been blamed for turning kids into drunken delinquents, I had approximately five hours to write a 1500-word feature on the ramifications of this war on lolly water.

My brain hurt as though I was hearing nails being scraped down a blackboard. I could barely keep my eyes open. The prospect of writing an intelligible treatise on Australia's horribly convoluted alcohol-taxation system — and the effective ban on a product that, at that point, made me gag just to think about — was unpalatable, to say the least. But I did it. I pulled out stats, compiled tables, and rang up contacts to get their opinion on this watershed moment in Australia's history of dependence on grog. I even quizzed the then health minister, Nicola Roxon, thankful that it was a telephone interview and she didn't have to suffer the impertinence of my morning-after breath.

The article would go on to be showcased by my editors as part of *The Age*'s submission to the Pacific Area Newspaper Publishers' Association Newspaper of the Year Awards, with a blurb on how my reports had highlighted the devastating consequences of Australia's binge-drinking culture. I read the piece again after the awards, and marvelled at how much sense it made, and how little evidence there was that I might still have been over the limit when I wrote it.

A few months later, I was shortlisted in the 2008 federal government–sponsored National Drug and Alcohol Awards. I ended up being a joint winner, along with reporters at the *Geelong Advertiser*, which had run a brilliant campaign against drunken violence. I took to the lectern at Melbourne's Regent Theatre and made a brief speech, expressing my gratitude to the people in the sector who worked so tirelessly to turn around Australia's alcohol problem: people without whom I'd have nothing to write about. As I spoke — squinting in the stage lights and looking out at the 500-strong audience as the screen behind me filled with a giant image of my face beside a headline that screamed 'STOP THIS MADNESS' — I felt it: the cold, wet wallop of hypocrisy. I might not be getting stretchered into the back of an ambulance or carted off in a police car every weekend, but I sure as hell wasn't the poster child for the moderation movement.

But the only thing I knew with more certainty than the truth of my own hypocrisy was that as soon as I was off that stage I'd be diving headfirst into the nearest bottle of wine. I knew I'd get drunk; I knew I'd be hung-over the next day. It was a Friday night, and I'd just had a major win. When you win, you celebrate. And when you celebrate, you drink. Those are the rules. Who was I to argue with several centuries of tradition?

IT TAKES THREE years, several dozen more stories, and a whole lot of drinking before I hit the wall. Consigning New Year's Day 2011 to the expanding archive of days I'd rather forget, I wake up on 2 January hoping to feel better. I don't. I feel anxious, lost, and still horribly hung-over, my faith in the healing properties of a quarter-pounder meal and a chocolate-fudge sundae seemingly misplaced. It's past 11 o'clock on Sunday morning, but I'm far from ready to say hello to it. The sun, glinting through a chink in my bedroom blinds, seems to point at me, an outstretched finger of light challenging me to get out of bed. I shrink away from it. The memories of yesterday linger. My heart, while not quite galloping, is still cantering along as if it has somewhere really important to be. There's a sickness in my stomach, the origins of which stretch far beyond my New Year's Eve blowout. Anxiety jangles in my bones as I begin to acknowledge the obvious: drinking brought me here. And I've been here too long.

I start thinking about *Hello Sunday Morning* and what it would mean to give up alcohol for three months, turning over the implications in my head, trying to find an angle from which the prospect will look less absurd. It terrifies me — but that's how I know I have to do it. Yet I have many misgivings. How can I survive summer? All those warm nights with weekend barbecues, after-work drinks in rooftop bars, and lazy afternoons in beer gardens. Then there's the not-insignificant matter of my 35th birthday at the end of March. I can't remember the last time I had a sober birthday. The prospect is laugh-out-loud ridiculous. Maybe I can do three months without drinking, but just stop a week early so I can get pissed on my birthday.

The decision is too enormous. I pull the doona over my head, which, on day two of the hangover from the fiery pits of hell, is still thumping like a state-of-the-art subwoofer. Perhaps I'll just stay in bed a bit longer. (This is often my solution to dilemmas that seem too hard — the adult equivalent of thumping your fists on the floor and yelling, 'It's sooooo unfair!')

My horizontal tantrum is interrupted by the ringing phone. I can see that it's Loretta, one of my closest friends and long-time drinking-partner-in-crime. She'd been living in Europe for nearly two years, and returned home to Melbourne in December, via a ten-day silent meditation retreat in an Indian ashram. After her alcohol-free vegan getaway, her senses were heightened, her insides were cleansed, she'd acquired a startling new level of mindfulness and, disappointingly for me, her drinking muscles had atrophied. The realignment of her chakras had turned her into a two-pot screamer, and I found it deeply unsettling. At a particularly raucous house party just before Christmas — at which my friends and I put in a marathon effort, kicking on from midday Sunday to five o'clock the following morning — I'd watched Loretta watching us. As it got to the pointy end of the night, and the drinking, singing, dancing, and general messiness ramped up, there she was, standing silently on the edge of the 20-strong group, nursing the same beer she'd had for hours, bewilderment written large on her face. It was the look you might expect of someone who'd been teleported from their lounge-room sofa to the surface of the moon.

She skipped the New Year's Eve parties and went to stay with her family in country New South Wales, working in her brother's pub instead of drinking her way into the next year. I remember getting a text around 2.00 a.m., wishing me a happy new year and telling me she was tucked up in bed with a cup of tea and a meditation book. At the party, as I sipped my tequila from a martini glass, we laughed at her newfound virtuousness, placing bets on how long it would last. Secretly, I was jealous.

This late morning, I let the phone ring for a long time before I'm ready to answer. Loretta knows me too well to be convinced that everything's just dandy when clearly it's not, so I don't even try. I tell her about the hangover that won't die, the baleful panic attack, the fact that I'm still in bed, and the monumental brain fuck I'm experiencing at the thought of not drinking for the rest of summer and a big chunk of autumn. She is, as she always is when I'm in danger of losing my shit, calm, tender, and practical. 'Sweet, you don't have to decide anything right now. You just have to get out of bed.'

So I do. I douse my face with cold water, brush my teeth, put my trainers on, and face the day. Even with sunglasses so big they cover half my face, the sunshine hurts. But as I walk around a glorious-looking Princes Park, blue sky overhead, the pain slowly subsides and my pace quickens. I start to enjoy the warmth on my skin and the effect it's having on my thoughts. I imagine how much more rewarding a morning like this would be if I could look at it without grimacing; if I could look at it before midday. In the grand scheme of things, three months isn't that long, right? It's less than 1 per cent of my life so far. What do I have to lose — other than horrendous hangovers, a beer belly, and the gaping hole in my pocket?

Later, as it dawns on me I won't taste wine again till round two of footy season, I begin to get scared. But underneath the apprehension, the decision feels right. I am sick, in every sense of the word, of being drunk. There's no novelty in it anymore. Every. Fucking. Weekend. Sobriety can't be any more boring than that. I want to know what life is like without my beer goggles. I want to be brave enough to do all the things I do on a big night out — meet new people, dance, chat up guys, be silly just for the sake of it — without the Dutch courage that alcohol gives me. Can I shift the perception, seemingly hard-wired into my sense of self, that fun comes with a glass in its hand? After years of writing stories that sought to hold government and industry to account for Australia's drinking problem, it's time to put myself under the same spotlight.

January

I BEGIN TO rebuild myself from the rubble and prepare for the alcohol-free journey ahead. I stock up on herbal teas, move the wine from the fridge to the back of my tallest cupboard, buy new gym gear, and start to imagine how a svelte and sprightly — and sober — me might look. I picture myself in three months' time, transformed into some sort of superhero, the newfound energy allowing me to leap over skyscrapers and shoot lightning bolts from my now-sparkling eyes. In this future world I am physically and mentally lighter, I have abs you can bounce lemons off, and I've perfected the sort of conversational skills that will make me a darling of the after-dinner circuit.

The first few alcohol-free days are actually quite fun. It's a whirlwind of exercise, wholesome meals, and the thrill of taking control of a situation that had been careering away from me like an empty shopping trolley down the face of Everest. I start writing a list of all the things I hope to achieve during my vacation from booze. This love of lists comes from my mum, who is never without a folded envelope or Post-it note filled with the scribble of her life's most immediate priorities. Like her, I've learned that there are few greater satisfactions than the sight of a fully scored-off list. Hangovers, with their side serve of procrastination, have seen me consign many a half-completed list to the bin. But this is a new dawn, a new day. There's no room for dispiriting bins of stationery.

On the latest list, which I distinguish from its predecessors by assigning it to fancy notepaper and entitling it 'The Big List of All Lists', I write down my goals. They range from the practical ('clean apartment properly'), to the energetic ('start running'), to the perilously overdue ('DO TAX RETURN!!!'), and the hopeful ('find love'). The list is three pages long: one page for every month of sobriety. The chaos that for too long has reigned over my world has no idea what kind of regimented shit is about to come down on its head.

But I don't write a list entry for what I think I'll gain most from this experiment — maybe because I'm not sure I want to find out. By staying sober for longer than I ever have in my adult life, I may be able to figure out how I got here. It may provide the key to knowing why being drunk is so hypnotically appealing that I've been doing it almost every weekend since I was a teenager. Why do I place so much value in getting off my face when the downsides have started to cause me such grief? What is it about our culture that makes drinking a social necessity? If I'm a product of my environment, what is happening in the countries, Scotland and Australia, that have shaped me. Eighty per cent of Australians surveyed in a 2010 study said that they think we're a nation with a drinking problem. How many of us are willing to put our hands up and say we're part of it? It may be confronting to answer some of these questions, but it doesn't stop me from feeling invigorated. I love a challenge.

Yet as I ready myself to change the habits of half a lifetime, I find that not everyone is convinced of my ability to transform. When I tell my editor, Gay, about the three-month abstinence plan, she smiles and says, 'That's good, that's really good, Jill. I'm sure you'll get there.' The arched eyebrow and voice raised half an octave suggest otherwise. She's seen me lead the charge on too many staff nights out to believe that I'm ready to give up my role as unofficial *Sunday Age* social secretary so readily. Journalism, with all the stress of meeting deadlines and the unsociable hours, lends itself well to a lush's lifestyle. We might not all be the foul-mouthed, emotionally dysfunctional boozehounds Hollywood suggests, but there are enough of us who are to elevate the depiction beyond mere stereotype. In this context, telling my editor I'm not going to drink for three months is something akin to Hugh Hefner announcing plans to join the priesthood.

Some friends are equally stunned by my decision. One is so shocked that she confesses to spilling a glass of champagne on the carpet when she reads my pledge on Facebook. Others are genuinely baffled: 'It's a bit extreme. Couldn't you just drink on weekends?' Many are supportive, commending my 'bravery' and promising to help keep me strong.

My family are behind me, although Dad's reaction is fairly predictable: 'You missed out the middle stage — moderation.' This is a variation on his favourite catchphrase, 'everything in moderation'. In my early drinking days back in Edinburgh, he'd trot it out with a shake of the head and a smile every time I'd roll out of bed at lunchtime complaining about a hangover, just to remind me that no-one forced the glass into my hand. I'd argue that if we were true to his maxim, moderation itself should be exercised in moderation; he was undeterred. A source of tremendous amusement for him was watching me and my older brother, Neil, as we reached our peak party years, hit the town, and then hit the soluble aspirin the next day. I think he teased us because it was a relief for him to discover that others in the family were human. For the 38 years that my parents were married (they divorced, painfully but amicably, in 2008), Dad never saw Mum hung-over. 'I don't do hangovers,' she still tells us to this day. They'd go out with friends, and Dad would have a couple of pints, perhaps a port nightcap, and he'd wake up with a dull headache and a queasy stomach. Mum could get stuck into a few glasses of wine, follow it up with a couple of single malts and a whisky liqueur, and the next day she'd be singing in the shower at 6.00 a.m. as if her bloodstream was somehow impenetrable to alcohol. It was very annoying.

I obviously haven't inherited Mum's constitution. But after pledging to go alcohol-free, hangovers are, for now, a thing of the past. When you're used to feeling dreadful a couple of mornings a week every week for as many years as you can remember, it's a novelty to wake up feeling rested and fresh.

The first sober weekend is glorious. On Sunday, I can't help but feel quietly smug as my friends complain about their mornings-after while I've already worked out at the gym, been to the supermarket, and done two loads of washing before lunchtime. Sobriety also gives me the time to read more and start writing again, filling pages with creative musings and bashing out the beginnings of short stories on my laptop. The early mornings are surprisingly enjoyable: the deserted streets, the sense of space — and the stillness. It's purifying. I feel like I've been let in on a well-guarded secret.

A week in, and I'm amazed at how easy this abstinence lark is. I thought I'd have been tempted by now, but the desire for alcohol has all but disappeared. Every day that passes leaves me with a stronger sense that my body and mind are cleaner than they've been in years.

After two weeks without alcohol, I feel great. My skin is brighter; I'm energised, happier, and fully committed to life as a responsible drinker. Mentally, it's as if a fog has lifted: my mind is clearer; my thoughts are more sharply focused. I'm calm and motivated at work. There are moments when I feel so alert and full of vigour that I fear I may burst into a round of star jumps. It's weird; I hadn't expected to take to sobriety so enthusiastically. I don't miss drinking at all.

TO UNPACK THE genesis of my booze-free odyssey, let me take you beyond Australian shores to discover how a binge-drinking Scottish hack came to be a binge-drinking health reporter 17,000 kilometres away from the chilly climes of her homeland. It started, as so many of these stories do, with a boy and a few drinks. It was the year 2000 — a date that seemed such a fanciful prospect during my childhood that when it finally arrived I was a bit disappointed not to be whizzing around on a jetpack and having my every whim catered to by a robot butler. In our third year at high school, five friends and I pledged that on the first day of the new millennium, wherever we were in the world and whatever we were doing, we'd return to our Edinburgh high school and have a reunion in the bike sheds, picking up where we left off: smoking fags, drinking cheap cider, and rocking out to Guns N' Roses' *Use Your Illusion II* on a beaten-up ghetto blaster.

I'm pretty sure that nobody turned up. The richly imagined future we saw for ourselves come the age of 23 turned out to be largely the same as our present, at 15. Most of us hadn't left the area — I was still living with my parents in the house I'd resided in since I was a baby — and our musical tastes hadn't expanded vastly. My taste in alcohol hadn't improved, either; I was still a cider girl. This was long before it became a boutique beverage for the inner-city crowd — I was a fan in its paint-stripper days. Diamond White, K cider, and Merrydown: these were drinks that packed a punch.

But I had expanded my travel horizons. After I graduated with a journalism degree, my friend Sharon and I hightailed it to New Zealand, where we spent a year backpacking and drinking our way around the South and North islands. We returned just before the turn of the millennium, and I landed my first job: as a reporter for a regional weekly paper just outside Edinburgh.

At the same time, I took on a part-time bar job, working Friday nights in Espionage, a new James Bond–themed nightclub. It was a cavernous labyrinth encasing five bars over four floors, starting at street level and burrowing deep into the bowels of Edinburgh's Old Town. It was also a building that cradled my past; between the ages of 16 and 19 it had been my second home. Back then it was called The Mission, and that was an appropriate name. I'm not religious, but I worshipped this place with all the fervour of a holy man, prostrating myself every weekend on a blackened altar of metal, grunge, and indie. With fake ID in one hand, vodka and Coke in the other, and dressed in Seattle-standard shorts over leggings, flannel shirts, and Doc Martens, my friends and I would lose ourselves in lyrics that spoke to our teen angst. Returning to work there in 2000 was the ultimate pilgrimage.

The club had a different air to it in its new incarnation. There were neon fridges filled with Bacardi Breezers where the cloakroom used to be, and the bouncers wore suits and earpieces instead of combat trousers and beanies. But the makeover didn't fool me: on each level I swear I could see sweat dripping down walls, and could smell patchouli oil and Red Stripe soaked into the sticky floor. I saw snapshots of my past in every corner. It might have undergone a slick facelift, with leather furniture and a lengthy cocktail list, but at its core still beat the heart of a grunge venue. But all those memories would be eclipsed when, in my old stomping ground, I met the man who would bring me to Melbourne.

His name was Hugh. He also worked behind the bar. When we first met and he told me that he was a backpacker from Tasmania, I must confess I wasn't immediately sure what nationality that made him. But I was sure of one thing — he was very cute. He had the sort of boyish smile and luminescent blue eyes that could loosen the knickers of a nun. He simply had to be my boyfriend.

On Valentine's Day 2000 I made my move. Fiona and I got pissed and went to Espionage, where we could get discounted drinks and I could eye up the cute Tasmanian barman. Hugh — who, fortunately for me, had broken up with his South African girlfriend the previous day — had no idea what was coming. My chat-up line, delivered with all the subtlety of a marching band at a séance, went something like this: 'The trouble with all you Aussie backpackers is you come here to see Scotland and all you do is hang out with other backpackers. YOOOU *[dramatic pause, wagging finger]* should be with a Scottish chick.' He politely said he was flattered, but that it was too soon after his break-up to contemplate a new relationship.

His romance ban didn't last long. We hooked up the next night after dancing to '70s funk at a dingy venue called Jaffa Cake, in the shadow of Edinburgh Castle. Never underestimate the seductive powers of a nightclub named after a chocolate biscuit, or the feminine wiles of a half-pissed Scottish chick with a plunging neckline and access to her mother's expansive collection of malt whiskies. And from this most unlikely of beginnings came an eight-year relationship that would take me to a life on the other side of the world.

When I arrived in Melbourne in the winter of 2001, I felt right at home in a country that not only had an international reputation as a hard-drinking nation, but also seemed to celebrate it. If Scotland were a man, he'd be wearing a kilt and sinking single-malt whisky by an open fire; Australia would be a larrikin in board shorts and thongs, chugging beer at a backyard barbecue. Language barrier aside, I suspect they'd be good mates. In those first few months, I think I heard about cricket star David 'Boonie' Boon's legendary 52-can in-flight beer-sculling record more times than I heard the national anthem. And what other country can boast a prime minister who entered the *Guinness Book of World Records* for downing a yard of ale in 11 seconds — an achievement that Bob Hawke believes may have won him more votes than any of his policies. This was the land of the drive-through bottle shop, the birthplace of the esky. I was in heaven.

A contact who had previously worked in the Melbourne office

of a Canadian company once told me that she realised just how internationally renowned Australia was for boozing when the firm introduced a no-alcohol policy: management declared they would no longer buy booze for staff consumption at work events. The company had been sued in Canada, by the wife of an employee who had died after drink-driving following a staff function. But its offices in Sydney and Melbourne were exempt from the booze ban. The executives told staff: 'Alcohol is so engrained in the Australian culture and way of life that we will make an exception.'

It may be the Aussie way of life, but it seems that this culture has turned toxic. In the ten years since I first set foot in this wonderful sunburnt country, concern about alcohol problems has intensified, growing with every year that passes. Public drunkenness and violence on city streets are hard to ignore; underage drinking is rife. The fallout from this boozed-up lifestyle is devastating. Emergency departments are filled with casualties — in an average week, 57 Australians die and 1500 end up in hospital as a result of excessive drinking. Rates of alcohol-related crime, violence, and chronic disease have soared. That burden, added to healthcare expenses and loss of productivity, costs the economy $36 billion a year.

So how did Australia get here? Is this just the way it's always been in the 'lucky country'? And if it is, what's driving this culture? If I want to know how I got here, hung-over and thoroughly sick of it, perhaps I need to understand how the heavy drinking culture that's nurtured my way of life was formed. When I first stopped drinking, some friends told me proudly that Australia sits at the top of the heap in world drinking ranks; I should be embracing booze, not turning my back on it. One colleague went further, saying that it was 'un-Australian' to swear off the grog: 'It's part of our heritage. It's who we are.'

I wonder if that's true, or if it's just a convenient story we tell ourselves to explain our love of the bottle. Three weeks into my booze ban, I seek answers to these questions by drawing on the research of one of the world's leading alcohol-policy experts. During the five years I've written about these concerns, he's been my go-to research man, a veritable guru of booze. Professor Robin Room, director of the Centre for Alcohol Policy Research at Turning Point Alcohol and Drug Centre in Melbourne, has been working in the field for more than 40 years. He says that a reputation for heavy drinking is part of Australia's 'national myth'; it fits into a romantic self-portrait of a country of rugged bushmen, who tell tall tales and share drinks with mates after a hard day's yakka. This is the equivalent of America's Wild West mythology — a gang of miscreants thumbing their noses at polite society.

But the reality is a bit more nuanced, according to Room. Just as I learned to drink in Scotland, Australia's early culture of heavy drinking was transported from British shores. In the 18th century, a gin epidemic swept through Britain and Ireland, causing devastating social problems and a mass crime wave. By the late 1700s, jails were overflowing and the first convicts were sent to Australia, with a penal colony established in 1788 in what is now Sydney. When teetotaller Captain William Bligh became the fourth governor of New South Wales in 1806, he saw drunkenness as a problem among the wealthy New South Wales Corps, who ran the colony and had a monopoly on trading rum. Bligh banned the use of rum as currency. What followed was one of the most dramatic uprisings in Australia's history. On 26 January 1808, about 400 Corps members, wielding bayonets, marched up Sydney's Bridge Street to Government House and declared martial law, placing Bligh under house arrest. It became known as the Rum Rebellion, planting in the national consciousness the idea that fighting for the right to drink alcohol was a key part of Australia's cultural identity.

Yet historians argue that the rebellion had little to do with rum, and instead was the culmination of a long and complex power struggle between Bligh, who wanted to control the way the colony was run, and settlers such as John Macarthur, who headed the Corps and wanted more freedom, including the unrestricted right to own property. The name 'Rum Rebellion' was actually coined 50 years later, by a teetotaller called William Howitt, who liked the alliteration and wanted to further the belief that the colony was awash with booze.

Popular folklore suggests that early settlers brought more alcohol than food with them when they first arrived. The belief is that they then got sozzled regularly, drinking more grog per head of population than any other country in the world. But this, says Room, doesn't withstand scrutiny. While they did drink heavily — about 13.6 litres of pure alcohol per person per year — the level of consumption was not markedly different from that of other countries at the time. 'In those early years of the colony in Sydney, the consumption per capita was high, but once you accounted for the fact there weren't many children and women around, it wasn't that different from Britain, and it was actually less than the United States at that point,' Room says.

Heavy drinking *was* rife during the gold-rush period of the 1850s, as masses of men were thrown together without the influence of women to tame their excesses. Itinerant bush workers, sheep shearers, drovers, and stockmen who toiled in the Outback also drank a lot, which helped to give rise to the concept of 'mateship'. I'd never heard this term until I moved to Australia, but it immediately appealed to me, this idea that the nation works most cohesively when you offer friendship and loyalty to your fellow countryman, whether they're a mate, a stranger, or even an enemy. In the early 19th century, this notion, at the core of the fledgling national identity, was linked closely to drinking. Workers rewarded themselves with collective alcohol binges at the end of a hard week's slog — an early incarnation of the 'work hard, play hard' concept. It also gave rise to the custom of 'shouting', in which men would take turns buying a round of drinks for their mates.

There were more women and children in Australia by the late 19th century, and men increasingly moved from the bush to the suburbs. Consumption dropped to 5.8 litres of pure alcohol per person per year (about half the levels of early colonial days). Beer began to be favoured over spirits. Room says that from this point, Australia had a Jekyll-and-Hyde attitude to drinking. On one hand, there was the notion of male bonding and mateship, which relied so heavily on alcohol; on the other, there was the rise of a church-led temperance movement. This latter was in part a reaction to high levels of public drunkenness and violence in cities, as more hotels and taverns opened up — much like we're seeing in modern-day Australian cities. The movement also gained popularity with women's groups and working-class men, who saw the harm that hard drinking caused. They wanted a better life for their families, and fought to reduce alcohol consumption, lobbying to have licences restricted and closing hours moved back.

But as the temperance movement gained dominance, an anti-temperance culture began to take hold among the bohemia: writers and artists who viewed the war against booze as a puritanical outrage. Led by Sydney's *Bulletin* magazine, the notion of the 'wowser' — a joyless meddler trying to restrict the freedoms of the masses — was born. I'd never come across this Australian term when I arrived, but I quickly learned that it had deep cultural significance. As Room tells me, 'The caricature of the "wowser" as a thin, hawk-nosed puritan, dressed in black and bearing a rolled umbrella, perfected by *The Bulletin*'s gifted cartoonists, has left an indelible image on the Australian consciousness.'

To this day, being branded a wowser is seen as an affront. The fear of being portrayed as that sticky-beaked prig means that politicians discussing restrictions on the sale or promotion of alcohol will often preface their comments with the disclaimer 'I'm not a wowser ...'. Nobody trusts a non-drinker.

Perhaps this goes a way to explaining why some people have reacted so defensively to my decision to give up booze. It's only been three weeks, but already some are treating my abstinence as if it's a personal insult. At a party during my second week of non-drinking, I was asked, 'Don't drink, don't smoke — what do you do?' My identity was suddenly reduced to the sum of the substances I'd chosen not to ingest. Despite repeatedly telling the host that I was driving, he insisted that I have a cold beer to toast the birthday boy, his brother. 'C'aaarn, y'can have one. Just one. C'aaarn, just one beer. It's a party!' Eventually I had to tell him I'd necked a couple of whiskies before I left the house, just to get him to leave me alone.

Alcohol loosens us up. The implication is that you're an uptight control freak if you abstain. But the suspicion of teetotallers is also scorched onto the Australian national psyche, the mistrust stretching all the way back to the days when non-drinkers were viewed as religious killjoys intent on curbing civil liberties.

The temperance movement scored its biggest victory during World War I, when six o'clock closing for hotels and taverns was introduced in four of the six Australian states. The idea was to cut down on drinking hours to encourage men to spend less time in the pub and more time with their families. The unfortunate consequence of that legislation was what became known as 'the six o'clock swill': men would finish work at 5.00 p.m. and race to the nearest pub to drink as much as they could in that last hour before closing. Chairs, tables, stools, billiard tables, and dartboards — anything taking up space that could otherwise be filled by drinkers — were removed from the floor and walls to allow for the fast flow of booze. Hotels lost their friendly feel and became hostile environments crammed with drunk, aggressive men jostling for service at the bar. Women were all but banned. With opening hours slashed, the continued temperance push, and the post-war Depression, alcohol consumption fell to its lowest levels during the 1930s, to just 2.5 litres per person.

Once in place, six o'clock closing proved hard to repeal. Despite its increasing unsavouriness, referendums proposing a move to ten o'clock closing were resoundingly defeated, in New South Wales in 1947 and Victoria in 1956. But public opinion finally swung in the other direction, with the move to later closing coming to New South Wales in 1954 — and not until 1966 in Victoria. It's hard to reconcile the 24-hour drinking culture of the Melbourne I know with a city that until relatively recently had such strict rules around booze. It doesn't fit with the presumption that alcohol has always been at the centre of Australian life. However, with early closing repealed, drinking gradually shifted from being the sole domain of men to becoming a more social pastime involving the whole community. Women began to be integrated into the drinking culture, as hotels were allowed to serve alcohol with meals, and sports clubs were granted liquor licences, turning them into social hubs.

What followed was an increase in drinking that peaked in 1975 at 13.1 litres of alcohol per person — levels not seen since early colonial days. This shift away from Australia's puritanical past was felt most keenly in Victoria in the 1980s, when premier John Cain set about turning Melbourne into a continental-style all-night city with a thriving bar culture. Since 1984, there's been a four-fold increase in the number of places where you can buy alcohol in Victoria. Deregulation in the 1990s relaxed liquor-licensing laws, leading to a proliferation of quirky laneway bars and cocktail dens. But it's also had a significant downside. For alcohol researchers such as Room, the consequences of this unfettered growth of the night-time economy were inevitable: as the number of late-night venues has grown, alcohol-related violence, injuries, and accidents have skyrocketed. He says that politicians — spooked by the spectre of wowserism and by a cashed-up liquor industry that aggressively pushes the free-market ideology — have been reluctant to take measurable legislative action.

Interestingly, at the same time as licensing was being deregulated, Australia was at the forefront of tough drink-driving laws. In 1976, Victoria became one of the first jurisdictions in the world to introduce random breath-testing. By 1988, the practice had been adopted nationally. 'That certainly went against this whole cultural frame of Australians as big drinkers. But the way in which it happened — there was a trade-off going on,' Room says. 'They did away with early closing in pubs, but brought in more restrictions on drink-driving. They justified the tightening up of one area by liberalisation in another.'

In a country where the tyranny of distance made driving home from the pub standard practice, particularly in the bush, these laws helped to shift that culture. As road accidents and fatalities came down, so too did alcohol consumption, dropping to about ten litres per person (over the age of 15) in the early 1990s. Rates have remained fairly steady ever since.

So, despite what some of my friends have told me, by world standards Australia is not the nation of champion drinkers that legend suggests. According to a World Health Organization report released this year, Australia came in at number 30 of 180 countries, lagging behind Nigeria, South Korea, Uganda, the Seychelles, and many countries in Europe, including Ireland, France, Germany, and the United Kingdom. Drinking everyone under the table with a whopping 18.22 litres of alcohol per head was the tiny Eastern European republic of Moldova. Any self-respecting Aussie beer-guzzler would be embarrassed by that.

It seems the story of the nation's drinking culture is a little more complex than the 'this is who we are and who we've always been' narrative. Room accepts that, historically, there have been cultural links between national identity and drinking, and that overall consumption rates are not markedly different from — and, in some cases, are significantly lower than — those in previous eras. What worries him and others in the public-health field is that many of those who *are* drinking are doing so at increasingly harmful levels. He believes that the rise in binge drinking we're witnessing, particularly among young people, is not tied to some romantic notion of the larrikin Aussie beer-lover, but has been manufactured by a market that treats alcohol as if it were a commodity as benign as tea or butter. Booze is readily available on every street corner, in shopping centres and drive-through bottle shops, and in pubs and hotels at all times of the day and night. It's cheaper and more widely advertised than ever before. Australia has also moved from a beer-drinking nation to a country of wine lovers, leading to a wine glut that has seen prices plummet and problem drinking increase.

'The politically safe line for doing something about our alcohol problems is to say, "We've got to change the drinking culture," because saying that means it's a longer-term project than happening next week. And secondly, it becomes almost code for saying, "We'll leave the market alone,"' Room tells me. 'It's an alternative to saying, "Why the hell do we have places that sell alcohol at five in the morning? Why do we let the supermarket chains sell alcohol so cheaply?" The fact that alcohol is available at more hours of the day than would have been true of any time after World War I in Australia — that's an issue. The way that countries find their way out of these periodic binges is through a mixture of regulatory action and changing the culture. If you think about what happened with drink-driving, it wasn't simply a matter of, "We've got to change the culture of people thinking they can get in a car after they've had a few drinks." There was also a tough regulatory edge to it.'

After chatting to Room, I'm heartened that I can place my own drinking habits in the context of a 'periodic binge' — a boozy blip in history, if you like. I'm sure if I'd reached adulthood in the temperance era I'd have been much more restrained. But what happens beyond the binge? For me, the answer will come in two months: I'll either go back to old habits or I won't. For Australia, a country where getting hammered is seen as a birthright, the end point is less clear.

AS JANUARY DRAWS to a close, my productivity continues to improve. I find that there are more hours in the day when I'm not drinking. But although I'm still enjoying feeling alert and healthy, the initial glow of sobriety is starting to lose its sheen. Saying no is getting harder.

The summer sun throws up some tough moments. A 40-degree day watching my friends drink chilled sangria in the pool while I sip water. After-work drinks with colleagues in a riverside beer garden — them: a bottle of sauvignon blanc; me: organic lemonade. I feel as if I'm missing out, and find myself resenting that I can't join in. When I committed to stop drinking, I pledged I wouldn't hide; I was going to go out just as much and have just as much fun as I would if I was drinking. But after nearly a month without alcohol, I'm not sure that's possible. I'm still going out, but I've now become fixated on the fact I'm not drinking, positive that my friends are having a better experience than me. I've convinced myself anew that sobriety is boring.

Then comes the night that changes everything. Cherry Bar is a rocking little live-music venue down a grungy city alleyway, cranking out kick-arse tunes till dawn. It's a Melbourne gem, and one of my favourite places to lose myself in an indulgent swirl of music, dancing, beer, and — occasionally — questionable blokes. One of the owners is a friend: James Young, a rock 'n' roll showman who successfully lobbied the council to have the laneway renamed AC/DC Lane in homage to the iconic band's Victorian roots, and whose parties are legendary. This night, Australia Day eve, is his birthday bash. The combination of a bunch of my closest mates, great music, and a bar serving free beer and Jägermeister shots is going to be a huge challenge. For the first time, I question whether I'll be able to resist temptation.

An hour in, and my apprehension is palpable. I can't stop looking at my watch, trying to gauge whether the clock really does tick faster when it's powered by booze. On a big night, it's not unusual for my friends and me to spend five or six hours at Cherry. Surely I'll get bored without the blurring of time that alcohol creates.

As I drink my soda water and lime, watching my friends knock back free beer, I tell myself I'll give it another hour before I make my excuses and drive home. I feel horribly exposed without a drink in my hand. The more I focus on my difference, the more self-conscious I become, tucking hair behind my ears as my eyes dart around the room. Little things that I would usually be oblivious to start to grate: the way my boots stick to the tacky floor, the smell of spilled beer, and the thin line of sweat forming on my top lip.

I retreat to the toilet to have a word with myself. Being sober is not the problem; my fixating on it is. So I decide to stop. I head back out and start enjoying the music and my friends' company, rather than worrying about where the night will go.

My friend Tash's boyfriend, Andy, who affectionately calls me 'Rockin' Jill' (a tribute to my energetic style of dancing) is concerned that without beer I will rock no more. By 10.00 p.m., his fears prove unfounded. When I hit the dance floor, something extraordinary happens — my whole body buzzes, arms and legs blissfully ignoring the voice in my head crowing, 'You can't dance sober.' I'm no longer the social pariah; I'm once again Starkers, the party girl. Jumping around like a teenager, it suddenly seems so obvious: it's not pints of beer or Jäger shots that make a night special; it's good music, great company, feeling loved, and the sense of confidence you project when those elements align. That feeling you get when a band belts out a chorus that makes it impossible to sit still is not exclusive to being drunk. The rush you feel when a favourite singer hits a note that wraps around your heart and leaves you breathless is just as real when you're drinking water.

This is truly a revelation. Big nights out on the piss have been part of my life for so long that I couldn't imagine what a night like this would look like without alcohol. Now I know. It looks clearer and the feelings last longer. Without alcohol fraying the edges of my memory, the experience is more profound. Perhaps the sweetest moment of the night is hearing one of my oldest friends and awesome dancing partner, Amy, tell me that sober Jill is just as much fun as drunk Jill.

There are testing moments tonight too, of course. There's the young man who sidles up and asks, 'What's your name, darl?' despite the fact we met ten minutes earlier, when he told me that I had the same name as his mother. Discovering that I'm Scottish, he becomes agitated when I can't tell him whether I'm 'on the IRA's side or the other lot'. (I later spot him on stage shirtless, wrapped in a curtain, head-banging to a Ramones number.) Having to constantly repeat myself also becomes frustrating as the night progresses, as does the tendency for drunk people to talk way too close to my face. Is there always this much projectile spittle, and I'm usually just too boozed to notice?

But there's a bigger epiphany to come. It's so unexpected that I'm completely blindsided. This night, I bust my long-held belief that alcohol is an essential element in any romantic connection. He's a friend of a friend; he's hot. There's chatting. There's dancing. There's a kiss. And then several more kisses. I can't remember the last time this happened without the assistance of alcohol. Admittedly, I'm more self-conscious than normal, my eyes flickering open to see if anyone's watching, but I guess that's natural when you're pashing the face off a virtual stranger in a public place, aided only by soda water. Without the fuzziness of beer, I'm much more aware of where

I am and what I'm doing. I'm in the moment — and the moment is pretty good. My words are honest and considered, not delivered in a nervous jumble of expectation and awkwardness. I don't know if that's what sparks the connection, but I know that I feel more confident and attractive than I would if I was slurring my words and slamming down tequila shots.

Contrary to my preconceptions, sobriety is not a man-repellent. He finds it fascinating, asking lots of questions and commending my fortitude. Halfway through the evening, he even switches to water in solidarity. Later, he walks me to my car, asks for my number, and kisses me good night. If only all of my evenings at Cherry Bar had ended in such a civilised fashion. As I drive home at 2.30 a.m. — a peculiarity in itself for someone used to being poured into a taxi at the end of a night — ears ringing, brain still buzzing, I smile when I realise that tomorrow there will be no hangover.

February

MY CHERRY BAR awakening is a turning point. I start to question every belief that I hold about the role of alcohol in my life. I've always thought that drinking gives me confidence; that without it I'd be a shrunken version of my alcohol-inspired alter ego. But if I can carve up the dance floor, party till the wee small hours, and pick up a cute guy without touching a drop, what else can I do sober?

Suddenly I see it: the emperor is wearing no clothes. For so long, I thought that alcohol gave me my edge, and the courage to speak my mind: a flick of the tap, and I'm served up a cold glass of liquid confidence. But often, this unfiltered honesty gets me into trouble. Such as the now-legendary post-work drinks that saw me give my editor an hour-long masterclass on how she should run the paper. Or the time I confessed to my mum, over a bottle of wine, that the mysterious dent in the wall she'd been puzzling over for years was caused by an unexpectedly airborne television, thrown during a teenage party that briefly turned my parents' living room into a mosh pit. After one too many beverages, I can be reckless with the truth, hurling it at people indiscriminately. But I'm coming to realise that at the heart of many of these conversations is an unmet need — whether it's the need to express professional frustration, atone for

youthful misdeeds or, most commonly, to tell the people I care about
the most the things I dare to say the least. ('I love you, man. No,
seriously, I, like, really, really love you.') Beer as truth serum. Vodka
as emotional lubricant. Wine as aphrodisiac.

It's a beautiful thing when an introverted friend not comfortable
with public displays of emotion tells you, after a few cocktails,
that you make her world a brighter place. A personal story shared
in confidence over a glass of wine can be the moment a casual
acquaintance becomes a friend. It might not happen if you're
clinking glasses of water. But why is that? Besides the physiological
effect that alcohol has on inhibitions, it gives us a convenient safety
net, I think, should the recipient of our truth-telling not react in the
way we might like. If we make a move on someone and they don't
reciprocate, we can always say, 'It was the booze talking — sorry
about that.' If the new friend finds the outpouring of emotion lame,
we can laugh it off later, notching it up to drunken nonsense. It's a
get-out-of-jail card, and I have used it so many times.

If I have a difficult subject to broach with someone close to me,
I'll often consciously plan to bring it up three or four drinks into the
night. I figure that's how much alcohol it takes to give me the balls
to say it, and to hopefully loosen up the recipient of my pent-up
candour. In relationships, I've used booze to help raise problems that
are troubling me — and you don't have to be Dr Phil to work out
that's not a recipe for lasting love. One fledgling romance ended after
less than a month when, at the end of a night filled with fine dining
and flirting, I decided to bare my soul. My plan was to explain
delicately that I'd just come out of a long-term relationship, and was
scared of being hurt. But my words became mangled in alcohol's
spin cycle, and instead I demanded to know where the whole thing
was going, how serious he was, and what his intentions were for our
future. As he fled into the night, I was left with a wilting mojito, and
cartoon plumes of smoke where my beau once sat.

But I've not been rendered socially incompetent by removing beer from my life. Perhaps booze is just a placebo. We think it gives us confidence, so we feel confident. In fact, there's research to back up that theory. Several studies over the last 40 years have shown that, while alcohol undoubtedly has a chemical effect on motor performance, memory, coordination, and reaction time, social behaviour and mood changes may be influenced less by how many tequilas we knock back, and more by the expectations that we bring with us to the pub. In experiments, psychologists have shown that groups of people who were told they were drinking vodka started to display certain behaviours — for example, becoming more confident and flirtatious — even when they were only drinking tonic water. The results of these 'alcohol expectancies' experiments suggest that, just as I use booze as a truth serum, to spill my secrets and mouth off about my frustrations, people routinely use drinking as a way to behave in ways they otherwise wouldn't because they believe they're drunk.

If we Australians think that drinking makes us more attractive and dynamic, it's no wonder that so many of us can't get through the weekend without a glass of wine. These perceptions are formed from an early age. The way in which alcohol has been marketed — as if that cold beer is going to transform you from a nerdy, no-mates loser into a bronzed and shimmering demigod, fighting admirers off with a bull whip — creates the impression that booze is our social elixir. Without it, we'd be desperate, dateless, and alone. Many young Australians struggling with their identity and with trying to form relationships have learned that drinking is their ticket to belonging. In a 2008 study from the University of Wollongong, 90 per cent of 15- to 24-year-olds who were shown a series of alcohol adverts said that they thought the products shown would help them to have a good time. More than two-thirds of the 300 high-school and university students interviewed felt that drinking would make them more confident, sociable, and outgoing, while 70 per cent said that it would help them to fit in. Half thought that the drinks in the ads — which included Tiger beer, and the liqueurs Frangelico and Kahlua — would help them to succeed with the opposite sex; almost 60 per cent thought it would make them less nervous.

These perceptions have not arisen by accident. As part of a 2009 inquiry into the conduct of the alcohol industry in the United Kingdom, the House of Commons Health Select Committee obtained internal marketing documents from a number of alcohol companies and their advertising agencies. One of the key findings from the documents was the importance that alcohol producers place on selling the notion that their brands can help to foster a sense of togetherness. Internal planning documents for Carling, a leading beer brand, described it as a 'social glue', stating that 'owning' sociability was the way to dominate the booze market. This was borne out by the commercial for its 'Belong' campaign, which featured a flock of starlings re-creating the word 'belong' in the style of the Carling logo. The internal documents stated that the campaign 'celebrates, initiates and promotes the togetherness of the pack, their passions and their pint because Carling understands that things are better together'. Documents obtained for the same inquiry found that the brand promise for Lambrini, a sparkling pear-based drink that comes in a range of flavours, was that 'it's the perfect social lubricant', and would 'make you and the girls forget your dull working week and transform you into the glamour pusses you know you should be'.

The industry in Australia is no different. You only have to look at the website of one of the country's largest beer companies to see that alcohol is being spruiked as a social necessity, and as the panacea for all our woes. An advert by Carlton & United Breweries, which makes Carlton Draught, Victoria Bitter, and Crown Lager, shows a young, attractive man walking into a bar full of similarly good-looking drinkers, and claims that 'communities are strengthened through the unique, everyday bonds our beer creates'. In video footage that shows the man laughing and bonding with friends and family, the voiceover tells us:

> We're there for the little moments where people feel comfortable with who they are and who they're with and we understand that what we make has always and will always be right there in the thick of things as people create friendships, face adversity and enjoy prosperity — from the casual beer at the local to grandest of celebrations, to the moment where you just want to drop back home to remember where you came from and where you belong. In fact, we believe, in a society becoming too busy to pause for simple pleasures, if a whole lot more people raised a beer in friendship, the world would be a better place.

Yep, that's right, we can heal the world with beer. Perhaps all that's required to achieve peace in the Middle East is a few dozen slabs of VB and a tray of party pies. After all, alcohol can help us to make friends, cope with tough times, celebrate victories, and generally improve our otherwise sad and dull lives.

Until very recently, I'd have said the same thing. Now, I'm starting to think that there might be a more constructive way to express my emotions or to make new connections. It won't always be easy, but I want to be honest with the people in my life, without having to be drunk to do it. When I tell my friends and family I love them, I don't want there to be any doubt about why I'm saying it. If I'm frustrated at work, I'd like to find a way to communicate my grievances in a manner that might actually get me the desired result. If I'm attracted to someone, I don't want to wait until I've had a skinful to tell them. It might be scary laying myself bare completely sober, but it's got to be more authentic than dipping the truth in a bottle of wine and calling it real.

HABIT IS A peculiar beast: she's not easily tamed, and she's not afraid of a dare. My body might be learning that I don't need alcohol to feel good, but my brain is following a more familiar script. As I attempt to order a lime and soda in a bar with friends one night, I'm shocked to hear the words 'vodka, lime, and soda' come out of my mouth, nearly sabotaging my booze ban just weeks after it's started. When I correct myself, the barman asks why I'm not drinking.

'A social experiment,' I reply.

He looks at me quizzically. 'Why on earth would you want to do that?'

Five minutes later, he approaches our table, sets down a shot glass, and says, 'We've just got this new vodka in. It's beautiful, really smooth, goes perfectly with lime and soda. I'll just leave that with you.' Smirking, he walks off, leaving us staring in bemusement at this strange offering.

Twenty years on the piss and all I had to do to get free alcohol was renounce drinking?

He returns ten minutes later, taking the untouched vodka shot with him. 'Well done — you've passed the challenge.'

I didn't realise I was being tested.

It's the first of many occasions where my decision not to drink is taken as an open invitation to try to knock me off the wagon. I'd like to think that my personality hasn't been muted because I'm not drinking booze, and that I can still crack a joke and hold up my end of a conversation, but some people are intent on proving me wrong. 'When can you drink again?' they ask with panicked voices, as if my life is on hold and any endearing character traits have abandoned me.

Sometimes I wonder if people would be more relaxed if I were holding a beer bottle. Even if it were filled with water, I suspect that the illusion would be enough to ease their tension. I'm starting to realise that even if I don't need alcohol to enjoy social situations, sometimes it makes other people more comfortable if I act as if I do.

Melbourne radio host Derryn Hinch — a former heavy drinker who gave up alcohol for health reasons — says that non-drinkers in Australia are marginalised and ridiculed. 'I've had friends who've gone to pubs, and I'll say, "I'll have a lemon squash." They'll say, "Why? You're a girl!" A female says, "I'm not drinking." "Are you pregnant? Is there something we should know about?" The non-drinkers are [treated like] criminals,' he told a conference on alcohol-related brain injuries in 2008. In my second month of sobriety, the truth of that is bearing down on me with great force. Like non-smokers at an office party in the 1970s, teetotallers are the new social pariahs. Being sober in a nation where 80 per cent of people over the age of 14 are drinkers feels like being part of an underground counterculture you're not sure you asked to join. That historical fear of the wowser is so engrained that I can only imagine how tedious it must be for people who never drink to have to face this level of pressure and mistrust on a regular basis. It's tiring to constantly explain why you're not drinking, in a culture that does little to embrace a booze-free lifestyle and much to encourage the opposite.

So I decide to ask one of the only non-drinkers I know how he copes with a life of permanent sobriety. Nick is my friend Bridget's husband. He grew up in Canberra, where the two met in high school. Being around him is easy; he's a natural conversationalist who will always make you think and often make you laugh. He's a full-time entertainer, performing stand-up comedy, magic, and conman tricks for corporate clients and pub crowds. I've never asked why he doesn't drink, but I've always wondered. Today, over lunch in a Northcote cafe, he tells me. 'I started drinking when I was about 17, the usual house parties where everyone goes along and drinks too much. There's a history of alcoholism in my family, and I have a really addictive personality, so I would come home from school and have a beer by myself. All day I'd be like, I've got to get home and have a beer; I've got to get home and have a beer. I didn't really notice it was a problem until I was about 18 and my girlfriend died in a car accident, and that knocked me about a bit, so I started binge drinking. I'd get paralytically drunk all the time. I'd drink every day. Then I just realised I can't be a person who drinks.'

Eighteen months after having his first drink, he stopped. Not one drop of alcohol has passed his lips since. A self-confessed control freak, he won't even nibble a rum ball at Christmas or eat food that's been flambéed. The pressure to drink, he says, is enormous and unrelenting. But it hasn't come from the people he expected. His teenage friends had no problem when he quit drinking. Neither do the working-class men for whom he now performs, in tough pubs in Melbourne's western suburbs. It's people in suits who give him the hardest time. 'I feel like I could do a lot better in business if I drank. I have corporate functions where everyone goes for a beer, and people want to chat to me afterwards and buy me a drink. I can say, "I never drink when I'm working," but after the gig's finished, I don't have an excuse. Not drinking makes me slightly removed from the event in a professional sense. I often say, "I might just have a Coke." It creates this weird tension.'

I'm becoming very familiar with that tension. Sometimes it's so uncomfortable I almost feel like apologising to the drinkers in my company. I ask Nick why he thinks people are so disarmed by non-drinkers. 'It's like they think, you've made a life decision that I don't understand, and I worry about what's behind that. It's kind of like if someone has a very different political opinion from me — if, say, they're pro-life — I'm always a bit like, "What's behind that culturally, because in my head I'm seeing you bomb abortion clinics," which is entirely unfair and untrue, but I think it's the same with alcohol.

'It's the thing that if two people go through a terrible experience together, they've shown a soft side; they've been through a war, and now they've bonded. It's the same with alcohol: "Well, we've been drunk together, we've lowered our inhibitions." It's that thing about the reason you shake hands is to show that you don't have a knife in your hand. Alcohol's a social lubricant. You say things you might regret later on, so if you're prepared to drink with someone, you're saying, "I'm prepared to let the real me out."'

I can relate to this. By choosing not to drink, it feels as if I have unwittingly broken a contract to be disinhibited. I have welched on that tacit agreement between drinkers to be candid, open, and in some ways vulnerable. When this contract is broken, it can turn ugly.

Nick says that celebrations, as I discovered with the beer-peddling birthday-party host, are particularly fraught. 'Weddings are tough. They bring out the worst in people when it comes to alcohol. People would give me champagne, and I'd say, "Sorry, I don't drink." "But it's for the toast. You have to have a drink." They want everyone to drink: "We are here to celebrate, you will celebrate, and we'll force this celebration down your throat in the way we want you to celebrate it." Everyone has to have a glass to drink, and it gets quite nasty.'

How will I cope with that sort of pressure? How will I get through my own birthday with a non-alcoholic toast? If I'm to survive three months of this, I'll have to start stockpiling excuses. I ask Nick for advice. He tells me that it's important to always have a glass in your hand. That way, if someone asks if you want a drink, you can simply say, 'No, I'm good, thanks.'

Also, I'm warned never to say, 'I'm not drinking' or 'I don't drink', as this only invites discussion as to why not, and immediately there's a barrier where there needn't be one. 'Just say, "No, thank you," and stare them down. "Go on, have a drink." "No, thank you." "Are you sure?" "No, thank you." And just ride out the five-second awkward pause,' Nick explains. 'I used to tell people early on that I was an alcoholic. I don't think I actually was because I did just say, "I'm going to stop drinking," and then stop. But I'd tell people, "I'm an alcoholic," and they'd say, "Oh, sorry," and back away.'

I like Nick's style. I've already been asked at least a dozen times why I'm not drinking. I can usually tell by the delivery where those who ask place on a scale that ranges from genuinely interested to obnoxious wanker, and I tailor my response accordingly. With that scale in mind, I formulate my own top-ten excuses for sobriety.

1. I just want to prove that I can do it.
2. My friends bet me I wouldn't last a month.
3. It's for charity.
4. I'm trying to lose weight.
5. I'm training for a marathon.
6. I've just come out of rehab.
7. NASA doesn't let its astronauts drink before shuttle launches.
8. My psychiatrist says I shouldn't drink on these pills.
9. Drinking makes the baby Jesus cry.
10. It's one of my parole conditions.

But I suspect that none of these justifications will suffice. It seems the only excuse you can proffer for not drinking that passes the 'you can have just one' test, other than Nick's 'I'm an alcoholic' line, is to say that you're pregnant. Anything short of being up the duff is open to negotiation. I start to envy pregnant women, who can happily turn down a drink without feeling as though they're altering the group dynamic or breaking a social contract. Theirs is seen as a decision of necessity, not choice, and therefore they're off the hook.

When I decided to stop drinking, I knew it would be tough, but I thought it would be a simple proposition of abstaining from the act of consuming alcohol. I wasn't prepared for the complex moral maze I'd have to navigate along the way.

A DECADE HAS passed since I came to Australia for what was meant to be a year-long working holiday, and turned into a life I never got round to leaving. Much has changed since then. My relationship ended, I got my dream job, and I bought an apartment, anchoring myself to a city I'd once known only through the slice of vanilla suburbia portrayed in *Neighbours*. I've seen friends and jobs come and go, and my clothes and hairstyle have changed, yet the one constant — other than taxes, the love of my family, and the rising and setting of the sun — has been alcohol. Wherever I've been and whoever I've been with, I have enjoyed getting drunk, regularly and unquestioningly. Drinking is the international language of social cohesion. When I was backpacking around Australia and New Zealand, it was drinking games that broke the ice with fellow travellers. In almost every job I've had, work friendships have been sealed in the pub. Getting pissed is how we bond with friends old and new, not just on the night itself but also the morning after.

On the tram one morning, I overhear a couple of guys in their early twenties talking about the previous night's adventures.

'I was wasted, man. I can't even remember getting home,' says one, who's wearing a cap low over a pair of mirrored sunglasses.

'How the fuck did I end up on top of that car?' the other asks.

Giggling, they try to retrace their evening, fitting their patchy memories together like a jigsaw puzzle.

It's a conversation I've had with many mates over many years. Big nights out are something we revel in, comparing the sizes of our hangovers and the fogginess of our memories over laughs and cups of tea in the staff kitchen come Monday morning. When you get drunk with friends, it's like taking a road trip together, destination unknown. You only need to look at the success of the *Hangover* movie franchise to see that there's a universal narrative about the unpredictable adventures that can arise through the common bond forged by drinking. We might not all have woken up to find Mike Tyson's tiger in our hotel bathroom, or pulled our own tooth out after marrying a Vegas stripper, but most of us will have at least one shared drunken escapade that we can recite proudly as proof that we've lived. Who hasn't woken up groggy and aching, with only a phone number scribbled on a beer mat, a half-eaten kebab, and a smudged ink stamp on the inside of their wrist as clues to the previous evening's events?

Deciding not to drink when your friends are still having these adventures is a bit like watching them go for a joyride in a Maserati while you're desperately trying to keep up on a skateboard. As the second month of my sobriety continues, it seems that no matter how hard I try to get a seat in the car, there's just no room. It's subtle at first, but slowly things begin to change. A couple of times, people arrange to meet up at the pub for a few drinks, and I only hear about it days later. I think they presume that if I can't drink, I won't want to be there; I'm not sure if this says more about their company or mine. When I *am* invited, they raise their glasses to cheers the group, but don't clink mine because it's filled with water. Without booze, it feels like I'm becoming invisible, paling into the background like a cloud in a whitening sky. Some friends disappear altogether, alcohol seemingly the glue cementing our relationship.

Those who do stick around can't hide their puzzlement at my decision. My workmate Cam says to me in exasperation, 'When's this all going to stop, Starkers?' as if I've lost the capacity for rational thought.

I laugh and say, 'Who knows? Maybe I'll go a whole year and write a book about it. I could call it "My Year Without Booze".'

His response, lightning-quick, floors me: 'Yeah, then you could write a sequel and call it "My Year With No Mates".'

I force a laugh. He means no malice, but the comment really bothers me. Am I committing a slow form of social suicide? If this is what people are saying to my face, what are they saying when I'm not around?

My abstinence is becoming such a focal point that I'm tired of talking about it. It's become my defining characteristic. I know that people are only bringing it up because they're interested, but it serves to underscore my difference, my otherness. I start to feel an affinity with vegetarians and vegans, who must face these questions of exclusion daily. I'm conflicted, oscillating between enjoying the positive physical and mental effects of sobriety and yearning to belong, in a way I haven't experienced since I was an angst-ridden teenager, pretending to like nosebleed techno in a bid not to be shunned by my peers. But I'm 34 — I'm old enough to know better. Certainly old enough to feel secure in my choices and confident of my place in a group, regardless of what I'm pouring into my glass. How hard must it be for younger people to walk this path? When you're in high school or at university, how do you opt out of a ritual so deeply engrained in society's collective sense of identity without alienating yourself from the world around you?

A recent survey conducted by the Foundation for Alcohol Research and Education found that more than a third of all Australians drink alcohol to get drunk. That figure rises to more than 60 per cent in Generation-Y drinkers. Interestingly, 37 per cent of those drinkers said that they'd tried to cut down their drinking and failed. It makes me wonder if some young people are getting pissed not because they enjoy it, but because it's easier than living life on the friendship fringe.

This was the case for a young guy I interviewed a few years back. Steve was a promising junior footballer who started drinking at 15 — the average age at which Australians have their first drink — and quickly became known as a party animal. He loved having a few beers; it helped him to relax. Friends said that he was hilarious when drunk. But he soon found that he couldn't socialise without it. He knew that he was drinking too much, but when he left school and enrolled at the University of Melbourne, where boozy parties and pub crawls were non-negotiable hallmarks of campus life, things began to escalate. It took 18 months of heavy drinking — his daily fix was a five-litre cask of wine and a six-pack of beer — before he could no longer cope and had to quit his studies. This perceived failure set off a chain of events that started with him crashing his car while five times over the limit, and ended with an overdose of antidepressants and sleeping pills.

What shocked me most about Steve's story was not the detail of his deterioration, but the fact that he started out just like me. 'I was just a normal teenager playing football, having fun with my mates, and drinking a bit at parties,' he told me. 'There's strong peer pressure; it's socially expected. If you don't drink, you feel a bit on the outer. It's really hard to go out and socialise if everyone's drinking and you're not.'

I'm not suggesting that every binge-drinking teenager is on a path to destruction, but as someone trying to stay sober in a world obsessed with booze, I just wonder if Steve's story would have been different if the peer pressure to have another beer and be that fun guy at the party weren't so great.

As I try to redefine my place in my own social circles, what's most surprising is that the friends I thought would pressure me the most — the hard-drinking boys who can knock back beers like a war's coming — are the most supportive. My sobriety doesn't seem to threaten our friendship in the same way that it does with some of my female friends. I hear around the traps that a few girlfriends are expressing concern that my break from booze is a judgement on their drinking habits. Until recently, these friends and I have all drunk in a similar fashion: we enjoyed getting pissed, and we did it regularly. By opting out, it seems that I'm implying there's something wrong with their lifestyle. At first I find this a ludicrous argument — my decision not to drink is no more a judgement on them than a vegetarian friend's preference not to eat meat is a moral statement on my carnivorous choices. And how could I, the binge-drinking reporter involved in a long and steamy romance with booze, ever retreat to the moral high ground about anyone's alcohol consumption? The stakes were just getting too high for me. If others drink in the same way and don't wake up feeling like a worn-out dishrag, good luck to them.

It bothers me that I've offended some of my friends simply by choosing not to drink. More than that, it hurts that they don't seem to comprehend how hard it is to stay sober when everyone else is hoeing into the red wine and beer. But then I see it from their point of view — in my bid to be unflinchingly honest, I've been telling the world about all the situations in which I no longer need alcohol, and how my life is being more richly lived sober. My words are sincere, but I can see how my enthusiasm could be construed as pompous. In less than two months, I've gone from a kind of ageing Lindsay Lohan to an alcohol-free, clean-living convert. So I try to be more understanding, and remember that it wasn't too long ago I would have berated anyone who left a party before 2.00 a.m., and crossed the street to avoid someone spruiking the merits of life without booze.

I gain more of an insight into the way my sobriety affects my friends when I'm invited to Government House, the Victorian governor's residence, for a garden party. The event celebrates the 25th anniversary of a leading medical research institute. It's a glorious 30-degree day with blue skies. I take my friend Kath along as my guest. As we walk out onto the manicured lawns in our heels and summer frocks, I feel as if perhaps I've made it in Melbourne. With the string quartet playing under the marquee, and waiters passing round canapés to suited and booted VIPs, it's a delightful scene. The lemon squash I have to settle for is somewhat less befitting the occasion than the expensive champagne filling Kath's glass, but once I resign myself to this, I quickly get over it and enjoy the afternoon.

As the proceedings draw to a close, I turn to Kath — the only person I know who's happy when the temperature tops 40 degrees — and suggest that we go to a rooftop bar in the city to enjoy the rest of the evening sunshine. She seems reluctant. When pressed, she says it would be weird because I'm not drinking. I can't get my head around it. I vowed, when I started this challenge, that while sober I would do all the things I would ordinarily do if I was drinking — and going to a rooftop bar with Kath is exactly what I'd do in this situation. Yet it's not me who's calling last drinks.

'Am I different when I'm sober?' I ask her, genuinely puzzled by our predicament. 'Am I not as much fun?'

She looks at the floor, saying something that makes me realise my sobriety is going to involve much more than simply not drinking for three months: 'I just don't like the idea of being out of control when you're in control.'

I don't know what to say. I feel bad for both of us. But then I remember: it's that social contract. Her barriers are down; mine are still up. By not drinking while Kath is, I've upset the equilibrium. She feels unguarded and defenceless in the face of my sobriety. How could either of us relax, knowing that she feels uncomfortable and exposed?

In the end, we do go to a beer garden for more drinks. She has champagne, while I have ginger beer and lime. I think, at least I hope, she knows that I'm not scrutinising her every move, trying to detect a slurred word here or a stumbled step there. Still, despite going out of my way to adopt just the right level of nonchalance to obscure her discomfort, I don't think she fully relaxes until we meet up with a group of friends for dinner, several hours later. Watching her greet them in the restaurant is like seeing an exchange student return home to their family after months of living in a foreign land. Finally: people who speak her language.

I thought that not drinking was going to be hard for me. I never expected it to be hard for anyone else. But I can see that while being the only sober one in a group of drinkers has its challenges, it's even trickier when you're in a one-on-one situation. No matter how hard you try, it's like you can't tune into each other's frequency — it's as if you're trying to communicate underwater. In a group, that disconnection is dissipated by virtue of numbers. Yet when there are only two of you, it can be an immovable barrier.

It's only when I can no longer reach for a bottle that I realise how much my friendships rely on it. As another friend's world splinters into pieces with the end of her relationship, I feel as if I've let her down because I can't share her pain over a drink. Break-ups require expensive cocktails and soul-baring girls' nights out, but I can't even buy a glass of champagne and toast the start of a new chapter in her life. I feel useless. I begin to realise anew that there are few occasions, happy or otherwise, where I don't use alcohol to enhance my relationships.

A few days later, a colleague at work with whom I've recently become friendly tells me that she's leaving to take a job in Sydney. She remarks that she wishes she'd got to know me while I'd been drinking. What an odd statement, I think, but then have to admit that I feel the same: we've grown close, sharing pieces of our personal lives during tea breaks at work, but something is missing. I think back to previous friendships that graduated from work acquaintances to something more, and almost all of them took that next step in the pub or at a party, helped along by beers. There's something about that journey — the laughs, the silliness, the shared experience — that bonds you to each other. There it is again: that contract to be disinhibited, unsigned on my part, and blocking my path towards deeper friendships.

It's a disheartening thought, but perhaps some things are simply incompatible with sobriety.

March

AFTER TWO MONTHS without alcohol, I barely recognise myself. The settings where I'd ordinarily reach for the wine bottle or head to the bar no longer trigger the Pavlovian response they once did. I can go to a gig and not worry about queuing for beers — and about missing the band in the process. At dinner with friends, I'm much more engaged in the conversation, listening in a way I might not have, had I let booze fill in the blanks. And to my great surprise, I've lost two kilograms without even trying. Getting to the gym is a lot easier when you don't wake up feeling as if you've been mowed down by a freight train. The sluggishness that convinced me I couldn't run has vanished, and I can now hit the treadmill for 45 minutes at a time — a previously unimaginable feat.

My eating habits haven't changed. If anything, I'm eating more of the things I shouldn't, as compensation for denying myself alcohol. I've become intimately acquainted with every dessert menu within a ten-kilometre radius of my flat. At the servo next door, the staff nod their heads and look at each other knowingly as I skulk in each evening for my after-work chocolate bar.

Yet still the weight falls off. There's only one explanation: I was carrying a two-kilogram beer baby. Those clever marketing folks may have tried to convince us that 'low-carb' beer is the guilt-free alcoholic equivalent of Diet Coke, but clearly booze is a natural enemy to weight loss, whichever way you sell it. A big night of drinking, followed by a hangover that leaves you too sick to exercise, plus a day of stuffing your face with carbs and saturated fat, adds up to an unholy trinity of calories.

My stress levels have also dropped. My natural propensity to catastrophise about relatively insignificant events is diminishing. A bad day at work is now a mere blip on the radar, and I recover from setbacks much more quickly without hangovers, which tend to amplify insecurities and impair rational thinking. My emotions are no longer tossed around like a plastic bag in the wind. When I put the wine in my cupboard, my problems didn't go away, but they certainly became easier to manage.

I haven't felt this healthy for a long time. It makes me worry about what I was doing to my body before I took this break. Sometimes hangovers would bring not only a headache and a fuzzy brain, but also a stabbing pain in my side. My rudimentary understanding of these things, coupled with a quick Google search, suggests that it may have been a dehydrated kidney or a saturated liver working overtime to break down all the alcohol I'd poured into it. Whatever it was, it wasn't good. For a health reporter, it's staggering how little attention I've paid to my body's warning signals.

But I'm not sure that the average Australian would know much more than me about the health consequences of heavy drinking. Aussies might joke about their big nights out and say, 'Thank God the liver's the only vital organ that can regenerate.' But the risks of a boozed-up lifestyle go way beyond a soggy liver. Australia's increasing number of alcohol-related health problems are part of a worldwide trend. As a planet, we're downing more booze than ever before. The World Health Organization is so concerned about the upturn in risky drinking that in February, delegates met to develop a global strategy to reduce alcohol harm. A report released at the Geneva summit showed that underage drinking increased in 71 per cent of countries over the five years to 2008, while 80 per cent of nations have seen drinking among 18- to 25-year-olds rise. The meeting heard that alcohol kills 2.5 million people a year — that's 4 per cent of deaths worldwide attributable to booze — and is the world's third-largest risk factor for disease and disability. It's a causal factor in 60 types of diseases and injuries, and a component in 200 others. More people die from alcohol-related disease or injury than from HIV/AIDS, violence, or tuberculosis.

Yet, despite alcohol being a group-one carcinogen — meaning that it's known to cause cancer in humans, putting it in the same category as tobacco, asbestos, and ultraviolet radiation — most Australians are oblivious to the risk. Cancer Council research in Victoria shows that only 9 per cent of people are aware of the link between drinking and cancer. Unlike the graphic Quit campaigns for smoking, which highlight the health risks and shock many of us into stubbing out the fags each year, the public education adverts about alcohol are predominantly focused on violence and injury. That's despite the fact that 5 per cent of all cancers in Australia — more than 5000 every year — are directly related to alcohol. I wonder if, had there been more publicity about the health risks, I would have cut my drinking down a long time ago.

To find out exactly how big a risk I was taking, I speak to Craig Sinclair, director of the cancer education unit at Cancer Council Victoria. For a man who has dedicated his working life to public-health prevention programs, he's frustrated that the message about cancer risk doesn't seem to penetrate a nation of drinkers. 'Alcohol is very much engrained in the culture of our life. It's got a very high social acceptance. The vast majority of the population drink it and enjoy it in moderation, and there's a lot of positive associations when people think of alcohol. So unlike tobacco or other carcinogens like asbestos, where it's much easier to draw a line between positive and negative, it's far more difficult with alcohol because you're challenging enormous social norms,' he says.

Sinclair and his colleagues believe they've got a big task ahead in trying to make people realise it is not just their liver that's at risk from drinking. Cancers of the mouth, larynx, and oesophagus — areas with which alcohol makes direct contact — all have a strong link to drinking. Increasing evidence also shows a very strong link to bowel cancer in both men and women, and to breast cancer in women. In fact, I'm shocked by how strong that breast-cancer link is: an analysis that Sinclair co-authored, published this year in *The Medical Journal of Australia*, revealed that 2600 new cases of breast cancer in Australia every year are caused by drinking — that's one in five. Even one unit of alcohol a day increases a woman's risk of breast cancer by 10 per cent, and the combined effect of smoking and high alcohol consumption increases the cancer risk significantly. As an ex-smoker with a history of breast cancer on both sides of the family, I'm starting to view my two decades of binge drinking as a high-stakes game of poker. But how much does someone have to drink before they increase that risk? Are we talking a couple of glasses of wine a day, or a couple of bottles?

Sinclair says that while there's a direct dose–response connection between alcohol and cancer, the evidence around how much is too much is not as clear as it is with tobacco. 'At low levels — less than two standard drinks a day — the risk is still there, but it's very low. If women are drinking heavy levels from a young age and continue to do so through their adult life, they're going to be putting themselves at far more significant risk.'

Controversial National Health and Medical Research Council alcohol guidelines released in 2009 warned Australians, for the first time, that there was no 'safe' or 'risk-free' level of drinking. They also advised parents not to give their children, even older teenagers, alcohol. The guidelines — criticised by the alcohol industry and some in the health field as too conservative, and therefore likely to be ignored by the public — describe 'risky drinking' as more than four standard drinks in one sitting (about two-thirds of a bottle of wine).

If you go by the national guidelines, I used to drink a lot. By the standards of my circle of friends, I was fairly average. The guidelines tell me that people should aim for an average of no more than two standard drinks a day, with two alcohol-free days a week and no more than four drinks in any one sitting. An official standard drink is one 100ml glass of wine or a stubby of mid-strength beer. Given that most bars serve wine in 150ml glasses, and that a bottle of full-strength beer equates to 1.4 standard drinks, I was probably drinking more than double, or almost triple, the guideline limit on a Friday or Saturday night. It doesn't seem like a lot to me, but the evidence is there: drinking like that over a regular period significantly raises the lifetime risk of long-term medical conditions such as breast cancer and heart disease.

It's a confusing message, considering it wasn't that long ago doctors were spruiking the benefits of red wine, in moderation, to protect against heart disease. Now, the Heart Foundation and the World Health Organization warn against this, stating that a review of the evidence shows that the positive effects of red wine in reducing cardiovascular disease have been hugely overstated. The message from the public-health lobby today is simple: your safest bet is to not drink at all, particularly if you're a woman (as our risk of cancer from heavy drinking increases more quickly over a lifetime). There's also evidence to show that women are at greater risk of alcohol-related neurological damage, liver cirrhosis, and depression than men. Researchers believe that hormonal differences, and the way in which women metabolise alcohol — we have less water in our bodies than men, so alcohol becomes more concentrated in our bloodstreams — increases its toxicity and promotes disease. So, the longer I carry on the way I've been drinking, the more chance I have of developing a serious health problem.

As my birthday approaches, those thoughts are at the forefront of my mind. How long can I continue to drink as if I'm invincible? On 24 March, I will officially become middle-aged. It may be time to start treating my body a little less like an Ibiza nightclub and a bit more like a Buddhist temple. The thought of turning 35 is scary. I can't remember the last time I spent a birthday completely sober, but I'd hazard a guess that Madonna was still a virgin, and I was sporting acid-washed jeans and a spiral perm. Until now, I'd rarely contemplated not having a drink on my birthday. But I'm determined to see it in alcohol-free. Finishing up my sobriety stint a week early would be a cop-out.

I brace myself for my friends' reactions when they find out that I'm having a sober birthday. They might find it hard to accept, given it's an occasion that has historically provided them with such amusement. I talk to Fiona in Edinburgh, who reminds me of my 15th birthday party, which my parents allowed me to have at home, leaving my 18-year-old brother and his mates in charge. It got so out of control that Fiona's cousin, an off-duty police officer who happened to be driving past, pulled up and hammered on the door to see if we needed assistance. There were teenagers hanging out of every window, and piles of vomit forming a Hansel and Gretel–style trail from our front door, stretching halfway down the street. As I came to the door, Fiona's cousin peered over my shoulder to see my brother kicking a party guest down the stairs for trying to use one of Mum's crystal vases as a beer glass.

At my 16th, my friends and I were sipping peach schnapps and lemonade (because nothing says 'we're of legal drinking age' quite like a peach-schnapps spritzer) at a city-centre pizza restaurant when our meal was interrupted by the arrival of a police officer. He began questioning me about my age, looking at this group of ten girls who were all wearing so much makeup we looked like kids playing dress-up. As my bottom lip began to quiver, the policeman started to recite poetry. He took off his hat and plonked it on my head. The serenade finished with a kiss on my cheek. Only then did I spot my brother and his best mate on the other side of the restaurant, pissing themselves laughing, his birthday present to me clearly more of a gift to himself.

At my 25th, after a month-long detox diet of brown rice and vegetables, I re-established my relationship to alcohol with such fervour that I have virtually no memory of the evening from about 10.00 p.m. Two male friends were forced to prop me up, *Weekend at Bernie's*–style, to get me past the bouncers of a nightclub. Once inside, I hit the dance floor — literally — after a series of poorly executed can-can kicks saw me land flat on my back, miniskirt around my midriff, bottle of cider still in hand. A friend later told me that when I hit the deck, the thud was so loud there was an audible gasp from the crowd. But thanks to the anaesthetising powers of booze, I bounced to my feet, punching the air defiantly like Judd Nelson in the closing scene of *The Breakfast Club*.

Hitting my thirties didn't slow the tempo. Quiet Sunday-afternoon drinks for my 33rd birthday morphed into an unexpected 3.00 a.m. adventure involving Jägermeister shots, a bizarre solo dance routine — in which photos taken by my friend Mel would suggest I was channelling a baby albatross trying to fly — and a brief dalliance with a dreadlocked life coach who called himself 'Zulu'.

Birthdays are fun like that. Not only do you have an excuse for acting like an idiot, but also your friends actively encourage it. This is particularly the case if it's a big number, such as 18, 21, or 30: it's a green light for drunkenness and fuckwittery, and I've never missed an opportunity to take full advantage of it. This year, I'm not sure how I'll even mark the occasion without raising a glass. Perhaps my birthday won't be real until its significance is recognised by having a proper drink, and until then I'll be preserved, petrified like a mosquito in a lump of amber, fabulously 34 for all eternity.

Worse still, this year, more than ever, I feel the need for a drink to ease the pain of the ageing process. When I was growing up, I imagined that by now I'd be settled down with a husband and a couple of kids. Yet here I am, five years away from 40, with no partner; still drinking like that scrawny, carefree teenager of the '90s; and faced with the very real possibility that I might never be a mother. That's not necessarily a tragedy; I'm not even sure that I want children. I'm grateful for what I have, and, for the most part, I feel content with my life. But it doesn't stop the occasional twang of panic.

As my birthday edges closer, this panic begins to play me like a banjo. What if I do meet someone and feel those maternal instincts, but my biological clock has run out of batteries? Perhaps that's why I used to get drunk so often: maybe binge drinking is a way to dampen the fear of being alone. Am I pouring beer and wine into a void that would be better filled with love? Or maybe I still drink as though I'm a teenager because I just don't want to grow up. Am I Peta Pan?

One of the joys of singledom is that there are no limits. You're your own boss. But when it comes to drinking, that can also be a disadvantage. There's no partner to pack you into a taxi when you've gone a bit heavy on the happy juice; there are no babies to ensure that the need to grab some sleep ahead of a 2.00 a.m. feed outranks the temptation of that last drink. That's not to say that my married or partnered friends aren't big drinkers — but they're rarely the ones cranking out indie classics on a novelty guitar and sipping tequila from a martini glass at five in the morning. Being in a relationship doesn't stop you from getting drunk, but it tends to curb the more unsavoury excesses of drunkenness. When you're single, your amplifier goes up to 11. Now, with the elucidation of sobriety, I'm forced to ask myself if, just maybe, my reasons for binge drinking stretch beyond the pursuit of fun and begin to stray into overcompensation for being alone.

My situation isn't uncommon. Australian women are getting married later, if they marry at all, and they're having children later in life. We've got more disposable income and less responsibility than previous generations. It's a cocktail (pardon the pun) for guilt-free hedonism. Getting older no longer means that the party has to stop: more than a third (34 per cent) of Australian women aged 20 to 29 binge drink at least weekly or monthly, having more than five drinks in one sitting and placing themselves at increased risk of short-term harm, such as accident or injury.

I always figured that my drinking would slow down if and when I had kids. But having a baby might not necessarily change my boozy habits. One in five — 21 per cent of — women in my age group (30 to 39) are binge drinkers. It seems that, for many of us, the drinking habits we learn as teenagers and young women carry through into later life. Surely not all of those women are single, childless thrill-seekers. Some of them must be balancing family life with getting drunk on the weekends.

I ask friends and contacts who were party girls like me before children came along. Some say that the changes in their bodies have left them with a much lower tolerance to alcohol; even if they wanted to get wasted, they just don't have the constitution for it. Many found out the hard way that hangovers are not an option with young children who sleep to their own schedule, and pay scant regard to your need to lie in a darkened room with a box of painkillers and a cold compress on your head. Others say that the challenges of motherhood make that end-of-the-day drink more coveted than ever before.

My friend Catherine reckons that before she fell pregnant for the first time, she hadn't gone a day without a drink in ten years. The pregnancy was a surprise, albeit a welcome one, to her and her long-term partner, which made the lifestyle change an even tougher adjustment. 'I knew I drank a lot, but I didn't realise how much until I had to give it up. I gave up smoking as well, and I think my body went into toxic shock. It wasn't like I was getting absolutely wasted every night before I was pregnant, but it was pretty easy for me to drink four beers or most of a bottle of wine every night because your tolerance is so high. I always had in my head that when I got pregnant I'd stop all this.'

Catherine started having the occasional glass of wine after her daughter was born, but it was only a fraction of what she used to drink. Gradually, though, she found herself getting closer to 'Habitland'. 'It's like smoking — it's just so insidious. You think, I'll have a nice glass of wine because I haven't been drinking at all, and then you have another one. And, also, it is that wind-down when you've had a really shit day. The four or five o'clock mark is always the hardest part of the day: it's a bit of a downer time, a natural serotonin dip in the day. It's just nice to have a bit of a wind-down — it's like a knock-off from work.'

After having her second child, Catherine's drinking has again slowed down, but she reckons she's got a few parties left in her yet.

A work contact, a senior executive in the not-for-profit sector who asks not to be named, tells me that while she's not going out to clubs like she did before she started a family, her drinking habits haven't changed much. 'A lot of my friends are also working mums, and they're in reasonably high-pressured jobs. When we get home, having that six o'clock gin and tonic is our time,' she says. 'It's an instant release. It's not easy to go and meditate for half an hour, or go for a run, when you've got three screaming children all wanting your attention. Sharing a bottle of wine is something that you can do together as a couple that is quite simple, and helps you to relax and debrief after a long day. You look forward to it.'

For this Melbourne woman in her early forties, working full-time and coming home in the evening to feed, bath, and play with the kids — one of whom has a severe disability — the wind-down gin and tonic or glass of wine with her husband rarely stops at a solitary drink. She knows about the national drinking guidelines, but says those rules are unrealistic. 'Normal people don't do that. Normal people sit down and have a bottle of wine with their dinner, and that's four standard drinks each. It's not a stretch to go, "Oh jeez, we've finished that bottle, let's have another one."'

Her weekends, while not as wild as they once were, are still full. Functions, parties, and barbecues are always accompanied by alcohol. 'If your friendship group is the party, going-out, socialising group, it doesn't change because you get married and have kids. You don't say, "I'm going to settle down now and never have another drink." You're not going out to the pub and having 20 drinks, but you're sitting chatting and you're having probably eight drinks, easily, without batting an eyelid. And I'm not even the biggest drinker in my friendship group.'

Her consumption levels are similar to mine. Is it naive to think that getting older or becoming a mum might change my drinking habits? Reading some of the *Hello Sunday Morning* blog posts, it's clear that for every woman who drinks less after having children, there's another who has kept pace with her old ways. Meagan, a 37-year-old mum of two boys aged three and five, from Townsville, says that her days would be a lot tougher without 'magic wine o'clock'. I get in touch with her, and she tells me that juggling a part-time job and motherhood is harder than she'd ever imagined. 'People think [that in staying home with children] you've got it easy — what a lark! — but in reality when you're at home with two kids under three, you just watch how quickly they trash your house. There were days where I'd go to unpack the dishwasher, and in the time it took me to do that, they'd emptied a whole tube of toothpaste in the bathroom, and smeared it all over the sink and up the walls and over the mirror. Or I'd make the bed and see this trail of flour footprints throughout the house, and they'd tipped out a container of flour, and they're acting like it's snow, throwing it all around my kitchen. The hardest days are the days where you don't get a break. You're just cleaning and washing and feeding and trying to provide them with entertainment.'

Meagan's Friday-afternoon drinks with her husband became her sanctuary. He'd finish work early, and they'd park the kids in front of a DVD while they sat out on the verandah, sharing a bottle of wine. 'You'd think, thank God it's Friday, we've got through another week. That was our way of unwinding and relaxing.' The ritual quickly turned into a habit on Saturdays and Sundays as well; three o'clock marked the start of drinking time. Lunches with her girlfriends were also boozy occasions. 'We've all got small children, and we get together every couple of months, and for me that meant lots of wine and then coming home and having more wine, and sneaking out to have some ciggies by the pool, where the kids couldn't see me. I'd have two or three glasses of wine at lunch, and then we might go to another venue after lunch and have two or three more. I'd probably end up, over the course of the afternoon, having a full bottle of wine. Then I'd get home and have more. Initially it was a bit of a joke, and you'd be on Facebook the next day saying "ouchy" or "I had to ride the porcelain bus last night," but it started to get to a point where I got really sick from the hangovers.'

Like me, Meagan decided to take a break from drinking after one hangover too many. It was the day of her son's fifth birthday party. She'd spent months planning food, decorations, games, and goodie bags for the superhero-themed party, but she woke up 'shaking and grey'. The previous evening she'd dropped in to see a neighbour, with no intention of getting drunk. She only had three glasses of wine, but they were large ones. On an empty stomach, and with her petite 49-kilogram frame, they went straight to her head. 'When I have too much to drink, I'll often smoke as well, and that made it a lot worse. I was just slayed the next morning. I spent so much effort and time in planning this to be such a special day for him, and then I felt like shit that morning. I just thought, there's no way in a million years that last night was worth today. I was terribly ashamed about being hung-over. To me, it just showed that I had kind of lost control.'

My editor at work, who married and started a family relatively early, has long been fascinated by my drinking habits. She often asks me what I get out of staying up all night binge drinking, a term that seems to be shrouded in virtual quotation marks every time she uses it. Recently, she told her daughter Beth about my alcohol ban, describing the prolonged period of partying that preceded it.

'How old is Jill?' asked Beth, who, like many 19-year-olds, gets on the piss most weekends.

'She's nearly 35,' my editor replied.

'Gaawwd. Thirty-five?' Beth sighed. 'Am I still going to be doing this when I'm that old?'

Just as I presumed that I'd give up my heavy drinking when I settled down, Beth thinks that hitting her thirties will change her habits — as if some arbitrary line in the sand will magically appear, and wine and cocktails will begin to taste like drain water. The reality is, turning 35, getting married, or becoming a mother might not change anything if booze is, and always has been, at the centre of your social life. If I was the only 30-something woman I knew getting trashed at the weekend and cutting a solitary figure on the dance floor, it wouldn't be long before I questioned my lifestyle choices. If Meagan was bringing bottles of champagne to afternoon tea while the other mums enjoyed chai lattes, it might be awkward enough to prompt some self-reflection. As it is, we slip into the social norm so seamlessly that it takes a hangover of epic proportions to make a change.

For young mums, it's getting easier to have a family and keep drinking. Increasingly, pubs are seeing the economic benefits of attracting parents by having playgrounds and children's areas on the premises — and the Australian climate lends itself well to sitting in a beer garden and enjoying a few drinks while your kids play in a child-friendly space. If the kids are safe and happy, their parents relax, which means that they'll stay longer and drink more. Some bars are so keen to get families through the door that they're offering free children's meals and colouring-in books, and even jumping castles. Meagan says that some of the pubs in her area have face-painting and indoor kids' areas monitored by video cameras, so that parents can drink in the bar but still keep watch over their children.

The move is all part of a shift in our culture that has seen more women drinking than ever before. Since the end of the six o'clock swill, women have been integrated into a drinking culture that used to be the domain, primarily, of men. The industry was quick to respond to this social change, developing wine coolers and sweet-tasting, brightly coloured pre-mixed spirits in stubby-sized bottles, to appeal to women who didn't like drinking beer. The 'alcopop', as the latter became known, was a massive hit with girls and young women.

Some alcohol companies are now looking to mothers as the next growth market. Australian online parenting community *Real Mums* has its own wine club, with bottles delivered to your door. 'No more dragging the screaming toddler to the bottle shop and having people look down their nose at you!' the website reads.

And I wonder how long it will be before we start seeing brands like MommyJuice sold here. This American wine company targets busy mothers. The logo shows a woman cross-legged on a yoga mat, juggling a house, a laptop, a teddy bear, and kitchen utensils. 'Moms everywhere deserve a break,' the blurb reads. 'So tuck your kids into bed, sit down and have a glass of MommyJuice — because you deserve it!' The battle for the mommy dollar is so fierce in the United

States that a rival company, Mommy's Time Out ('we all know that being a mommy is a difficult job') recently tried to convince a court, unsuccessfully, that MommyJuice's use of the word 'mommy' to sell wine was a trademark infringement.

While I'm fairly certain that most of my friends with kids would rather eat their own eyeballs than be seen drinking a glass of MommyJuice, I don't doubt that there would be a market for such a product in Australia. The mother-of-two behind the wine — the name for which was inspired by her children, who used to say 'That's Mommy's juice!' whenever they saw wine glasses — says that it's no different from beer ads, which have for decades used sport as a way to attract men. I'm all for market diversification, but it troubles me that women are being targeted in this way. Is drinking really such an intrinsic part of motherhood that mums are being convinced they need a bottle of wine to survive it?

To Meagan's surprise, the opposite has proved true. Since she stopped drinking, managing small children has become a lot less stressful. 'I realise now that I cope a lot better without alcohol. It was adding another layer of stress, because you can't really deal with your emotions and the real issues if you've got a bit of an alcohol haze around you. There's always that low-level irritability, even if you're not hung-over.'

And what about those boozy girls' lunches? They've got to be hard for someone who described herself as 'the life and soul of the party'. 'I really worried that they were just not going to be fun. I thought that these good times were all tied up with alcohol, but I had the best time recently with my girlfriends. I laughed my head off, and they were laughing with me. I realised that I'm just a silly duffer and, whether I'm drinking or not, that's who I am, and [not drinking] doesn't make me any less fun or interesting to be around.'

This gives me hope as I prepare for my sober birthday celebrations. Maybe I can still have a wild time without booze — only this time, my antics will be remembered for quite different reasons from my prolific drinking talents. It will be the year that Starkers stayed sober, and surely the novelty of that will be enough to elevate it to a position in the annals of history that will match the notoriety of previous occasions.

WHEN THE BIG day comes, I'm one week away from three months without booze and, oddly enough, this scares me more than the thought of a beer-free birthday. I started out doubting I'd last the full three months and now, as the finish line approaches, I'm questioning whether it's long enough. I've gained insight into my motivations for drinking, but I'm not convinced that it's enough to change my relationship with alcohol fundamentally. I can see myself a few weeks down the track, hung-over and regretful, spiralling into a chaotic world of late nights and lost mornings, just like old times. I've learned that I don't need to drink to be confident, honest, or affectionate, but I wonder how quickly those lessons will be swept from my mind, like footprints beneath a rising tide, when I'm faced with a good bottle of red and a night without limits. I now know that the line I thought age or motherhood might someday draw under my binge drinking is written in pencil, not permanent marker. If I don't want to be waking up with the same wretched hangovers five or ten years from now, I'm going to have to work a bit harder at changing the way I drink.

Besides, I'm not sure I'm ready to give up feeling so healthy, calm, and motivated. Just like my liver, I feel as if my body and mind are regenerating. The cells are being replenished.

I have a strange sense that I'm standing at a crossroads. I could go back to Habitland, where Catherine found herself so soon after having children, or stay a while longer in Sobertown. There are so many other experiences I want to try without alcohol. Can I survive a Melbourne winter without red wine? Will watching footy be as much fun booze-free? Could six months without alcohol see me kicked out of the Press Club?

I decide that another three months off the booze just seems right. It feels like I've got a lot more to learn before I invite alcohol back into my life.

Neil and his wife, Ker, and my nieces, six-year-old Daisy and three-year-old Orla, arrive on the week of my birthday. I'm excited to tell them that I'm going for another three months without alcohol. It's such a pleasure to have them stay in my new apartment, and to show them around the city I've grown to love so much. They live in Singapore, having moved there from Edinburgh three years ago. I soon realise that, although I can't toast their arrival with a beer, sobriety is actually making my time with them more special. Being dive-bombed by two squealing Scottish monkeys at 6.30 a.m. is much more enjoyable when you're not feeling scratchy after drinking wine till midnight. And when I find myself running with my brother around Princes Park at seven o'clock on a Saturday morning, I can only marvel at how things have changed.

On the afternoon of my birthday party, which I hold in a beer garden just to make the challenge more real, I'm feeling happy but a wee bit nervous. I've invited a lot of people and have a few pre-party jitters. I'm anxious that people will show up and that the weather will hold out. Mostly, I'm just thrilled that my friends will get to meet my family, and my Scottish and Australian worlds will come together, putting my two halves in context for those who love me.

It turns out to be a perfect day. The sun shines all afternoon, the kids play, and my friends and family gel beautifully. The idea that having a drink in my hand will somehow make the occasion more rewarding suddenly seems silly. True, there are no singing policemen or dalliances with dreadlocked life coaches, but that's okay. This year, I have more than that: I have the energy to immerse myself completely in playing with my nieces, I have the lucidity to appreciate how heartfelt my brother's words are when he says he's proud of me and the life I've made for myself, and I have several moments of genuine, full-to-the-brim happiness — the kind so warm you could curl up and live in them — made even more profound by knowing that they're not in any way enhanced, stimulated, or manufactured by alcohol. It is joy in its purest form.

April

LAST NIGHT, AS I slid along the polished floorboards on my knees, rocking the air guitar to Bon Jovi, it occurred to me: I don't need alcohol to be ridiculous. For so long, booze has been my ticket to a world of silliness. I have danced on bar tops, belted out karaoke, and waltzed with stolen traffic cones, all under the protective cloak of drunkenness. But as I enter my fourth month without alcohol, I realise that I don't always need a beer in my hand to be silly.

Nowhere is this more apparent than at an '80s dance class. Without alcohol to amuse me, I'm open to almost any form of alternative entertainment — and this one's a beauty. On Thursday nights, instead of enjoying pre-weekend drinks at my local boozer, I've been getting kitted out in legwarmers, fluoro tights, and a headband, and heading to an inner-city dance studio to bust out moves to classics from the decade that style forgot. We've done Alice Cooper, the Pointer Sisters, Xanadu, and, last night, the captain of cock-rock himself, Jon Bon Jovi. This is not a class for those who take themselves too seriously. So I decided pretty early on to leave my hang-ups at the door, rolled up in a ball next to my sweaty ankle socks and my vanity.

It gets me wondering, as I swing my ponytail around my head and pump my power fist in the air, why have I spent so much of my life worried about what other people think? Why has it taken half a bottle of wine for me to lose the self-consciousness that seems to follow me everywhere, like a playground bully? The more I think about it, the more I see that it's not going to alter the course of my life irreparably if a stranger thinks that my bum looks big in my new gym shorts. If I flirt with someone at a party and they run for the door, it might be embarrassing, but it won't kill me; and there's unlikely to be any long-term ramifications from an uncoordinated dance routine or a dodgy note in a karaoke bar full of colleagues. As Mum's been telling me since I was old enough to take fright at the sight of a full-length mirror, people are generally far more interested in their own lives than they are about the size of my bum or the relative boofiness of my hair on any given day. Yet I have wasted countless hours worrying about looking stupid.

This is part of the appeal of being drunk — it frees you from the suffocating constraints of social conditioning. You're either so blind that you don't know or care how you look, or you're consumed by the giddy hubris of intoxication, which colours everything you do with that glowing hue of awesomeness. I must admit that I do miss the liberation of drunkenness; you have to work a lot harder to feel bulletproof when you're sober.

So I have a choice. I can either be socially reserved, using my sobriety as an excuse for timidity, or I can let go of my inhibitions and channel my inner piss-head, minus the booze. This is what I did in February, when I saw one of my favourite bands perform: Primal Scream were touring, in celebration of the 20th anniversary of their seminal album *Screamadelica*. Hearing the wonderfully dishevelled Bobby Gillespie chunter on about the good old days in his gruff Glaswegian accent, as the iconic images of one of the defining albums of my generation played in a psychedelic light show behind him, I was transported back to the heady heights of my teenage years. As the first glorious bars of 'Movin' On Up' rocked Melbourne's Forum

Theatre, it was the closest I'd felt to being pissed since I stopped drinking. The music was so exhilarating that I couldn't help but dance like no-one was watching. But someone was. A picture taken by one of the *Age* photographers captures me dancing with such divine abandon — eyes shut, singing loudly, sweaty hair flying in all directions — that it prompted my friend Beck to comment on Facebook: 'Holy sobriety. I didn't think a girl could roll like that going pure.' I'm learning that if I can lose myself in the moment, free of introspective bullshit, alcohol becomes superfluous.

But sobriety can't make every night top-notch. At a less than enjoyable party earlier this month, I found myself hankering for a beer. Crammed into a corner, shouting banal pleasantries to strangers above the sort of doof-doof music you hear on government anti-drugs adverts, I fantasised about how a few beers might make this party better. Then it occurred to me: sometimes a shit party is just a shit party, and no amount of booze will change that. If only I'd figured this out earlier, I'd have saved myself a lot of energy making small talk with obnoxious try-hards and hooking up with charmless narcissists. Previously, if I was having a shit time, I'd drink more; I reasoned that the faster I could get pissed, the better the night would get. It wasn't great logic, and it rarely worked.

There are, however, some things I've not yet learned to do sober. Sex and soda water have proven to be incompatible bedfellows. Apart from my Australia Day eve pash at Cherry Bar — a romantic interlude which, incidentally, fizzled out before it began — my love life has ground to a halt. When I pause to reflect on why this might be, I'm faced with a number of answers. Firstly, I realise that I haven't been sober during sex in years, probably not since my eight-year relationship ended in 2007. After the split, I threw myself into a series of unsatisfying flings and one-night stands, unions all signed in the sticky ink of pale ale and vodka. I met most of the men in a bar or at a party — which, as we all know, is the ideal starting point for any meaningful relationship. There was the hot police officer, who insisted on having the true-crime television show *The First 48* as the soundtrack to his performance, and tortured me the next morning by blasting out Cold Chisel songs as he drove me home in his Holden Commodore. Then there was the 20-something guy I picked up at 5.00 a.m., after deciding he was potential boyfriend material based solely on the observation that he was sexy and wearing a nice hat. In the harsh light of morning, I discovered that his hat was clearly designed to deflect attention from the fact that he didn't seem to own shoes. And how could I forget the romantic charmer who did the deed and waited until I fell asleep to flee, leaving me to believe, for the first few minutes of the next day, that I'd dreamed the entire unedifying experience.

If this is the calibre of men I'm hooking up with when drunk, perhaps it's better to be sober and celibate. The ugly insides of the handsome strangers I used to be attracted to are so much easier to spot now that I'm sober. Several times in the last few months, I've had guys chat me up, only to see them lose interest when they discover I'm not drinking. It's disappointing, but instructive — the kind of guy who needs a woman to be drunk before he can make his move is not much of a man.

This year, I'm going to have to change my tactics. If those *Sex and the City* gals are anything to go by, I won't need alcohol to pick up blokes: I'll find my guy easily by seductively perusing canned goods at the supermarket, or by pretending to shop for power tools in a hardware store. Perhaps I'll join one of those singles cookery classes, or adopt a dog to act as a man-magnet.

While sober dating scares the hell out of me, it's got to be better than drunken dating disasters of the past.

WHEN I TOLD my editor that I was giving up booze, she thought it would make a good feature for the paper. We weren't really sure how the piece would take shape, but we figured that an examination of Australia's drinking culture, told through the eyes of a binge-drinking health reporter during a break from booze, might hold some interest for our readers. Now, she's shocked to learn that I'm voluntarily opting to stay sober for another three months. She presumed, as I did, that when 1 April came along I'd have the drinks lined up on the bar, trumpets sounding and party poppers popping, as I counted down the last few seconds of sobriety and prepared to embrace my old pal Boozy McBooze-pants. Instead, I find myself writing a piece about my three months without alcohol, and how it has changed me so much that I'm extending my drinking ban until July. Outing myself as a massive booze hound in the national press was not part of my career plan, but this is exactly what I'm about to do.

The night before we go to print, I'm hunched over the news desk, staring at a printout of the next day's paper. There I am, dancing like a maniac at the Primal Scream gig, my toothy grin and wayward mane prominent above a 2500-word confessional about my binge-drinking ways. My editor laughs. 'I can't quite believe you're doing this,' she says, and I shoot her a look so panicked that it prompts her to rest a hand on my shoulder and tell me not to worry. It doesn't reassure me. Holy shit — what the fuck am I doing? Tomorrow my colleagues will read this. Health professionals who respect me, and know nothing of my party-girl side, will view me in a different light. In 12 years of journalism, I've never had something so personal published. Our job is to report the news, and occasionally to give our opinion on it, but rarely to become it.

The next morning I wake up early to grab the paper. My tale of drunken debauchery takes up an entire broadsheet page. My face beams back at me; it's huge. In a secondary picture, I'm captured grinning inanely, my head wedged between two large glasses of beer — somewhere a village is missing its idiot. This morning I'm cocooned inside my flat, the blinds drawn, but I feel as if I've invited the world into my living room. I am starkers, in body, mind, and moniker.

Then the text messages start. Friends reading my story in bed while contending with mammoth hangovers tell me that they found it inspiring; it's made them think about how much they drink, and why. The head of public affairs at one of Melbourne's major public hospitals messages me to say that he found the article courageous and life-affirming. On Facebook and Twitter, friends, acquaintances, colleagues, contacts, and complete strangers are talking about the story in terms that make my heart lilt and my cheeks redden.

It's not even lunchtime, and the article has become the most-read story on the *Age* website. Dozens of people leave comments. Reading them, I realise that this is not just my story — my love–hate square dance with alcohol is one that countless others are having, week after week. Many are desperate to find a new dance partner. Some comments are from women my age, caught in a cycle of partying that's no longer satisfying. Others are heartbreaking: a man talks of his alcoholic father, reduced to drinking methylated spirits after retirement left him without the financial means to accommodate his habit; the father had died three weeks ago, brain-damaged, broken, and too young. For some, my story was neither uplifting nor motivational. One reader says that she found the article sad — sad that my peers define me by my drinking, and sad that I was scared to be my true self. Another thinks that the problem is not alcohol, but my inability to say no and to respect myself. One says that a six-month period of sobriety last year was 'the most boring and depressing time of my life', and informs me, ironically, that booze bans are usually instituted by social bores. A number of teenagers relate to my experience, saying they feel pressured to drink in an environment that views abstinence as abnormal. Nothing I've ever written has had a response like this — it's like group therapy for binge drinkers. It suggests that this is a conversation worth having.

By the end of the day, more than 30 new bloggers have signed up to *Hello Sunday Morning*, most of them saying that they were inspired to give sobriety a go after reading my article. Looking at their posts, which are full of the trepidation that comes with that first step, I'm reminded of how far down this road I am: I'm reminded of how insurmountable three months without booze seemed back at the start, and how insignificant another three months feels now. As I go to sleep, my body feels warmed by a day like no other. My head spins as if I'm drunk. It is 100 days today since I last had a drink. Sobriety has never been more intoxicating.

WHEN I GET to work the next day, there are more emails from readers, friends, and contacts. Chris Raine calls, and tells me that the *Hello Sunday Morning* server is struggling to cope with the number of new sign-ups. Colleagues are messaging me, and stopping me in the stairwell with supportive words. It's great that people have connected with the story, but I'm mindful that it also revealed I was a party-hardened reprobate who verballed her boss while drunk, and used alcohol as both an aphrodisiac and an antiseptic. Under the glare of the *Age* cafeteria's down lights, I start to wonder if my loquacious confession was perhaps a case of oversharing. I worry even more when one colleague wishes me strength, and emails me the link to a 12-step recovery program.

Thoughts of rehab are quickly shelved when I get an email from a publisher. They read the article and loved it; they want to meet with me and discuss book ideas. I call Loretta in shock. As she squeals down the phone, an email arrives from another publisher. I hold my head in my hands. It feels heavy, as if it might roll off my shoulders. Writing a book is all I've wanted to do since I was a nerdy eight-year-old, lost in blissful oblivion with my nose buried in an Enid Blyton story. Who would have thought that getting pissed every weekend for most of my adult life might be the way that dream comes true?

Later, I get a call from Channel Nine. They want to fly Chris and me to Sydney the following week, to appear on the *Kerri-Anne* show. I have to stifle a giggle. I know that while my friends will be delighted my article has won me professional accolades and approaches from publishers, the achievement of being interviewed by the queen of daytime television will bring me the most kudos in their eyes. This is a woman so outrageously kitsch that she once persuaded a sitting prime minister to dance the rumba, and a federal treasurer to bust out the macarena, on national television. I immediately say yes.

During the week, Kerri-Anne's producer is in frequent contact. I'm told that the interview will largely be based on the content of my article, and will centre on the challenges faced by a binge drinker who takes a break from alcohol. Chris and I are advised that we'll be sent a series of questions, and that our answers will be provided to Kerri-Anne as 'background'; I'm not sure why this is necessary, but I'm happy enough to do it. Yet when I get the questions, alarm bells ring. One reads, 'When you were having a lonely evening at home with just a bottle of wine for company, did you ever feel ashamed?' They also want to know how many drinks I had a day, and whether I ever drank at work.

I call the producer. 'It sounds like you're trying to paint me as an alcoholic,' I explain. She tells me that's not the implication, and that these questions are just to help Kerri-Anne 'get across the issue'. I'm wary, but she's persistent. I tell her that some nights I might have had only a couple of beers or, if I stayed home, nothing at all. But, thinking back to the marathon midday-to-5.00-a.m. Christmas party last year, I say that on rare occasions I might have had, for instance, ten to 15 drinks over a long period. This, I later discover, was a mistake.

When I arrive at Channel Nine studios in Willoughby, on Sydney's north shore, I'm nervous. It's my first television appearance, and it's live. I at least look respectable after being made over by the hair and makeup department, but I worry about having a brain spasm and being rendered mute on national television. Conversely, Chris, who could talk under wet cement, is chilled. We're led through a rabbit warren of stairwells and corridors to Nine's basement studio, where we're miked up and ushered on set without further instruction. We're seated on a pastel couch under lights that make me squint. The camera is trained on Kerri-Anne, sitting opposite as she wraps up the previous segment. We're presuming she'll then throw to a commercial break, allowing her to introduce herself and put us at ease before we're on air. Instead, she begins introducing our segment. 'On a big night of partying, my next guest, Jill Stark, was drinking about 15 drinks a day ...'

Fifteen drinks a day? My mouth drops open, and a snort escapes. I spot my face contorting in the monitor opposite and realise, to my horror, that I'm on camera — the image of my dumbfounded face is at that moment being beamed live to the nation. I compose myself as she continues to tell her audience about why I quit drinking. 'After one too many hangovers and a few regretful alcohol-related incidents, she decided to turn her life around.'

The interview is a train wreck. She infers I was a booze-hag, calls me Irish, and asks if I had 'big issues' with alcohol; the implication is almost that I was sneaking gin in the toilets at work just to get through the morning. She introduces Chris as someone who 'wrote a blog', without offering any further information, and depicts him, too, as a problem drinker. But it's live television, so we keep smiling and try to bring her back to the point: that we live in a culture that makes not drinking increasingly difficult. We're no different from thousands of Australians our age. It's disappointing that she either doesn't accept this, or chooses to ignore it. Even more disappointing is the caption — 'Jill Stark, reformed alcoholic' — posted beneath a link to the video on the Channel Nine website the next day. When I call up to complain, the producer apologises, telling me it was a 'human error'. But it feels like a stitch-up.

In hindsight, I shouldn't have been surprised. It's not the first time I'd had this sort of reaction to my temporary abstinence. The assumption is that if you have to cut alcohol out completely, you must have a problem. This idea fails to take into account our culture's unrelenting social pressure to drink, and drink to excess.

Tellingly, as we left the set, Chris asked Kerri-Anne what it would take for her to stop drinking. She rolled her eyes theatrically, saying with a smile, 'Oh, there'd be manslaughter charges,' and proceeded to regale us with tales of the entertainment industry's proud tradition of heavy drinking. 'Work is my handbrake,' she said, with a forced laugh. The hypocrisy nearly choked me. But I smiled and said nothing. What would be the point? I was learning that although this drinking culture touches us all, not everyone's ready to own their part in it.

IT'S GOOD FRIDAY and I'm invited to a friend's place for dinner. I'm working through the Easter weekend, and have just knocked off. My four friends have been drinking beers all afternoon, and by the time I arrive, they're quite merry. It's a longer holiday weekend than usual, with Anzac Day falling on Easter Monday, making Tuesday a day off too. Everyone's in the holiday mood, and the vibe is super-chilled. But I'm not feeling it: I'm still carrying the tensions of the newsroom, and I have to work tomorrow. For the first time in a while, I really miss beer. I just want to be on the same plane as my mates.

Knowing that I can't drink, I opt for Plan B. There's a joint going around; I take a few puffs. It hits me immediately. I'm not a big dope smoker — I'll have the occasional joint if it's passed to me at a party, but that's all. It usually takes a while before I feel the effects, yet today I'm stoned off my face after the first few tokes. It's not a good feeling; my body's become so accustomed to being in control that it doesn't react well to this foreign substance. I feel sick and my head's spinning. It makes me realise that taking drugs to circumvent my sobriety is not a great idea. The whole point of taking a break from drinking is to find out what life's like in an unaltered state, so getting stoned feels like cheating.

In the taxi home, I see dozens of people streaming out of bars. I've never paid much attention before because I'm usually working, but it seems that the Easter holidays have become a major event in Australia's drinking calendar. The next day at work, I look up some figures. Data from Turning Point Alcohol and Drug Centre shows a huge spike in alcohol-related injuries, hospitalisations, and assaults on the day before the Good Friday holiday. The number of people hospitalised due to serious motor-vehicle accidents also peaks on this day, as people celebrate the start of the long weekend.

What's more dispiriting is that Anzac Day — a day to commemorate the Australians who gave their lives in battle — has also become an occasion to get plastered. The rate of ambulance attendances for people who have passed out from drinking, and the number of presentations to emergency departments for alcohol-related assaults, increases by 50 per cent on this day. The 24 hours before Anzac Day are also associated with a higher risk of traffic accidents for people under the age of 25.

Arguably, public holidays are always big drinking occasions — people who don't have to work the next day are more likely to over-indulge. But the association between drinking and a day to remember fallen war heroes has recently been fostered, or at least co-opted, by the alcohol industry. The most obvious example of that is the VB Raise A Glass Appeal. This Carlton & United Breweries campaign began in 2009, and encourages Australians to show their respect for fallen diggers by raising a glass of VB, and donating money to the Returned and Services League and to Legacy, which cares for the families of deceased and incapacitated veterans. The adverts, shown each year around Anzac Day, are designed to tug at the heartstrings. We hear from Bill, who reflects on his service in the navy during World War II. Sitting at home in his armchair, stroking black-and-white photographs, he talks about his mate Paddy, who was 'sent to God' when a plane hit them. The ad ends with a shot of Bill holding a beer as he gazes out the window, an empty chair next to him, overlaid with the words: 'Wherever you are, whatever you're drinking, raise a glass for our fallen mates.'

The campaign is unquestionably for a good cause, and has raised over $2.4 million since it began, with VB donating $1 million of that. CUB makes no money from the campaign, as 100 per cent of funds go directly to the RSL and Legacy. But you have to wonder about how much goodwill these adverts buy the brewing giant — to have your brand associated with helping Aussie diggers, the most enduring symbol of national pride, has got to be worth its weight in gold. And telling the public that they can show both patriotism and respect by drinking beer is marketing genius. Every time someone donates online or sees one of the adverts, they're exposed to VB branding. For the public, this perpetuates the notion that drinking not only makes you more Australian, but is also the way that we commemorate the casualties of war. When you knock back a beer on Anzac Day, you're doing it for your country.

Another advert from the series features General Peter Cosgrove, the former chief of the Australian Defence Force, sitting at the bar in a pub. 'There are many departed friends I'd love to be sharing a beer with at this time of memorial,' he says, before urging viewers to honour the soldiers' sacrifice by going to the campaign website. 'On behalf of all our fallen heroes and their families: cheers,' he concludes, raising a glass. Although Cosgrove retired in 2005, for many he is still one of the most recognisable defence leaders of recent years. I'd expect army chiefs to show respect for the dead, but I'm surprised that they'd get into bed with a beer company, good cause or not, when the defence force is struggling with a drinking culture that its own leaders admit is out of control.

The chief of army, Lieutenant-General Ken Gillespie, stated that in 2009, more Australian soldiers died from alcohol-related misadventure than in the war in Afghanistan. He declared that the drinking culture had been condoned, if not actively promoted, by the organisation's leadership; soldiers often saw heavy drinking as their reward after long tours overseas. They'd been living in confined conditions for months, often in fear for their lives, and by the time they got home, they felt they'd earned the right to unwind by drinking with their mates. The problem began in the post-Vietnam era, Gillespie said, when defence cuts sapped morale and the army's public image took a battering over perceived failings in Vietnam. As a result, the leadership, himself included, spent far too much time at the bar. In an email to commanders, Gillespie wrote that he was sick of seeing near-daily reports of soldiers being killed, injured, or arrested due to drunken bad behaviour. His comments were a wake-up call — this year, the defence force advertised for a team of alcohol and other drug coordinators to set up support programs for soldiers with substance-abuse problems.

It is not a new thing for soldiers to have a beer to unwind after the horrors of battle. The idea for the Raise A Glass campaign came from a photograph found in the old Victoria Brewery, which shows soldiers from the 2/1st Australian Machine Gun Battalion in Egypt in 1941 — the men have formed the letters 'V' and 'B' out of empty beer bottles. But there's a difference between kicking back with a couple of beers, and drinking so much that you injure yourself or a comrade. If even the army, a proud symbol of nationhood, has an alcohol problem, Australia's drinking culture could take a long time to change.

I've been offered a publishing deal. The book will be a tale of a whole year of sobriety. When I was offered the contract, my first thought was: I can't wait to tell my folks. My second was: I can't wait to get pissed and celebrate. It's going to take a while to recondition my brain not to reward myself with alcohol for all of life's triumphs. Instead, I celebrate with a lovely dinner in an expensive restaurant with some of my closest girlfriends. I raise my glass (mineral water) to theirs (pinot grigio) and toast the start of a new chapter.

My friend Jodie gives me a desk as I prepare for the writing process. It has good genes; it gave birth to her PhD. I buy a high-backed leather chair with padded seat and ergonomically designed arms. I buy expensive stationery, and place framed pictures of my family on the desk to gaze upon for inspiration. Everything's as I'd imagined it: the inner-city traffic hums outside my window, and the skyscrapers twinkle in the distance as darkness falls over fabulous Melbourne. But when I sit down to write, I'm blank. I'm gripped by interminably long periods of nothingness. Something's missing — I need a drink.

The irony, of requiring a glass of wine to write a book about the benefits of not drinking, isn't lost on me, but I can't help worrying that I have cauterised my creativity by removing alcohol from my life. History is replete with artists, musicians, and writers who relied on alcohol to expand their minds and enhance their creative talents. It was the drug of choice for many of the world's most celebrated writers. Welsh poet Dylan Thomas liked a drink — so much so that it killed him (he succumbed to alcohol poisoning in 1953, after downing 18 shots of whisky). William Faulkner, a gothic writer from America's Deep South, favoured the mint julep, a bourbon-based cocktail. Oscar Wilde's drink of choice was absinthe, a potent anise-flavoured spirit that was once banned for its apparently hallucinogenic properties. Wilde described it like this: 'The first stage is like ordinary drinking, the second when you begin to see monstrous and cruel things, but if you can persevere you will enter in upon the third stage where you see things that you want to see, wonderful, curious things.'

I wonder if my writing will be less wonderful without alcoholic assistance. I need advice from someone who knows. I contact Australian author and columnist John Birmingham, who wrote *He Died with a Felafel in His Hand*, a comic, semi-autobiographical novel about share-house living that became a cult classic and was made into a movie. On Twitter, he often spruiks the merits of a good drink as an accompaniment to writing. Sometimes, while on tour, he uploads pictures of the martini or whisky he's about to enjoy. His prolific drunken tweets have become a must-follow feed of profanity and comedic entertainment. Alcohol seems to be a fundamental pillar in his book-writing process, as evidenced by tweets such as this one: 'Superchilled vodka? Check. Dangerous stimulants? Check. Freshly shaved Playboy bunnies? Double check. OK. Looks like we got us a book plan.'

We've never met or spoken, but when I call him at his Brisbane home and introduce myself, he responds warmly: 'Maaate, what can I do for you?' I explain that I'm writing a book, and I'm worried that my creativity will be muzzled by my sobriety. He's a successful novelist who enjoys a drink — could he have done it completely straight? He tells me that *Felafel* was written in five weeks of 18- to 20-hour days, living on 'hot chips, whisky, and amphetamines': 'It was written largely under the influence because it was such a grotesque time pressure to get it done that I needed a way to keep myself up, so pills and booze was the way I did that, and specifically whisky. Beer just bloats you and you don't feel like [doing] anything; wine puts me to sleep, like a soporific effect; but whisky, I found, for some reason, fires me up at night. It's probably why they used to call it firewater. I know from long experience that if I have to work through until one, two, or three in the morning, the way to do that is to have my first whisky at about 11 o'clock at night. Not to get absolutely shit-faced because you'll just pass out eventually, but one whisky an hour, for some reason, acts as a stimulant for me and lets me go for a couple of extra hours.'

This isn't exactly the answer I was hoping for. But he assures me this is not his habitual writing practice. During the day, he only allows himself non-alcoholic liquid refreshments, such as green tea or iced water. 'In the natural course of events I don't drink at all, and if I'm going to take a drink in the evening, it's because I'm editing. There's something about editing — you're not relying on any creative centres of the brain; you're just going through what you've done previously. It's process work: you're looking at sentences, the rhythm of them, and it's almost like you're taking them apart like a motorcycle engine and trying to put it back together in a more efficient manner. Particularly if you're using the George Orwell rule of never use ten words when two will do. There's no poetry involved; it's just mechanics, and, in that sense, it's easily done with a drink in your hand.'

He advises me not to drink at all while I'm writing the book. Alcohol will make it harder for me to think clearly, and it won't enhance my writing. Contrary to what I fear, creativity needs clarity, not intoxication, he says. It's unexpected advice from an author who has written newspaper columns that are practically love letters to hard liquor. But there's an element of performance to that, he says. He's an entertainer, who plays up his public image as 'some sort of crazed beast'. And his drinking always occurs after his writing day is done. He blames Hunter S. Thompson — the creator of gonzo journalism, whose work was heavily coloured by his use of alcohol and hallucinogenic drugs — for creating the myth that good prose requires chemical assistance. 'I get young baby writers and journalists who want to meet me, and I'll do that a couple of times a year almost as a public service, and a number of them turn up with fucking six-packs and bags full of dope. They just want to get on it. And I have to say, "You're here to fucking work — and more importantly, I've got a meeting with my accountant and my agent this afternoon. I'm not doing this shit." Thompson has almost an iron hold over the imagination of a particular type of young writer. They just assume that they've got to do the same stuff. What they don't see is that, yeah, he was rat-shit while he had those adventures, but when he sat down to write, he did it completely fucking straight. And he would often rewrite a page 18 or 19 times to get it just right.'

As I wind up the interview, he reminds me that many of the great writers who relied heavily on alcohol ultimately ruined themselves by drinking — often through fear of failure. 'To sit down and decide to write a book is, in some ways, to take one step along the path to your eventual doom. It almost certainly isn't going to work for you, it almost certainly won't sell, and there are so many people who have gone down that path and it's destroyed them. You're putting down that first step yourself, you're embracing it — and to suddenly start drinking while you're doing it is to almost hurry yourself down that path.'

Well, if I am on a path to my eventual doom, at least it might take me longer to get there by not drinking. But as I look for non-alcoholic ways to fill the gap left by wine and beer, I realise that some substitutions aren't much better than booze. Instead of sitting down to write with a glass of pinot, I'm inhaling chocolate as if it were oxygen. It's turning into quite a problem. This isn't a couple-of-Tim-Tams-a-night kinda thing; I'm talking a sell-the-family-heirlooms-and-sew-your-stash-into-the-mattress type of habit. I had low-level dependency issues with the brown stuff before I stopped drinking, but now my addiction has morphed into a beast that won't be sated by anything less than a chocolate fountain hooked up to its veins. If I don't have chocolate every night, I get antsy.

Easter didn't help. By the end of the holiday weekend, I'd eaten my weight in foil-wrapped eggs and was in fear of developing a body shape to match. At first I told myself that this was my treat: a girl's got to have some pleasures in life. I don't drink, I don't smoke, I don't drink coffee, I don't do drugs — apart from that ill-considered joint over Easter, which, the next day, caused me to have the closest thing I've felt to a hangover in four months — and I've even managed to kick my two-can-a-day Diet Coke habit. Chocolate is my only guilty pleasure. But the 'treats' I'm mechanically shovelling into my mouth aren't rewarding anymore; it feels out of control, a bit like my drinking was just a few short months ago. The significance of that is something I'm not yet ready to explore.

As I start planning the book, and another eight months without alcohol, I ponder where it might take me. Will I, by year's end, have changed my relationship with booze so much that the mere thought of an amber ale will make me nauseated? Or will I plunge back in, as if the year off the piss never happened? I suspect that finding out is going to be a bumpy ride.

May

I'M SO SICK of soft drinks. I can't be held responsible for the safety of the next barman who serves me another glass of lime and soda. The world of non-alcoholic beverages, I'm discovering, is infinitely boring. Lime, water, and dreariness appear to be the core ingredients. Sure, if you go to one of Melbourne's trendy inner-north bars, you might be able to persuade a grumpy hipster to mix you up a mocktail made from hummingbird tears and the juice of Himalayan goji berries, but in your average boozer, it's slim pickings for the non-drinker. There are only so many lemonades or Diet Cokes you can have before you start to feel bloated, and sick to the stomach. If I try to match my friends beer for soft drink, I risk sending myself into a sugar- and caffeine-induced frenzy that will see me licking pub windows and barking at passing cars. Nobody wants to see that. Two sugary soft drinks are about my limit, and then I move on to water. But it makes shouting drinks very difficult, which is of course quite un-Australian.

At Cherry Rock, a laneway music festival held by Cherry Bar, I ask the bartender for a soda water. 'We don't have any,' he tells me tersely. 'Try the outside bar.' Fair enough — soda water's not very rock 'n' roll. I push my way through the crowd in AC/DC Lane, to a trestle table groaning under the weight of VB cans, and ask what booze-free beverages they have. The only option is a five-dollar can of Coke. I haven't drunk a full-sugar Coke for years, but maybe the ten teaspoons of fructose will give me a buzz — and if I'm lucky, I might feel just a teensy bit like I'm drunk. Most of the time I enjoy being sober, but the desire for the buzz of those first few beers is starting to creep up on me again. I'm beginning to wonder if the longer this challenge goes on, the more I'll hanker for those feelings.

The can of Coke doesn't do it for me: it gives me a headache and makes me feel sick. It seems that there's a real gap in the market for an entrepreneurial business that can come up with a range of tasty, alcohol-free drinks, and convince bars not only to sell them, but also to promote them as a sexy alternative to booze. As it stands, a sad glass of water with a wedge of lemon floating on top is not enough to entice people away from their frosty beer or full-bodied glass of wine. When I ask bar owners about the lack of choice, they say there's no demand for a wider range of non-alcoholic drinks. Then they usually remind me that serving alcohol is a pub's *raison d'être*. The inference is that I should stay at home or go to a cafe if I want to drink juice and hot chocolate. But cafes mostly shut by 5.00 p.m.; as a non-drinker, where do you go if you want to catch up with friends in the evening? Going for a drink in a pub isn't such an appealing option, when all my local has to offer, for example, is lemonade or tap water. Besides, publicans don't like it much when you drink nothing but water for four hours.

After doing some research, I discover that a sober social scene may actually be a money-spinner. In Ireland, alcohol-free nights at clubs in Dublin's Temple Bar pub district have taken off. One permanently alcohol-free nightclub, now in its third year, draws crowds of up to 400 a night, pulling in punters with a range of organic drinks, massages, face painting, and a cafe. It's proved so successful that the club's creator has expanded into Galway. Another sober night at a nearby dance club is thriving, offering its clientele, who are largely in their late twenties to early forties, smoothies, juices, and herbal teas. In Liverpool, a new venue that owners claim is Britain's first 'dry bar' is proving popular with a diverse crowd, including people battling drug and alcohol addiction, Muslims, and single women who want to enjoy a night out without being harassed by drunken yobbos.

If there's demand for non-drinking venues in Ireland (the birthplace of Guinness) and Liverpool (which has the highest rate of alcohol-related hospital admissions in Britain), there's surely a market here. I call the Victorian branch of the Australian Hotels Association, the industry body representing pubs, clubs, and hotels, and ask them if they know of any alcohol-free bars or club nights in Melbourne — and if not, if they think there would be demand for such a venue. The deputy chief executive, Paddy O'Sullivan, usually an affable chap, sounds annoyed. It doesn't make any sense, he says in a tone that suggests he thinks I may have gone slightly mad. 'I've been trying to get my head around it, and in an Australian context, running a pub that doesn't actually serve beer or liquor sounds rather odd, actually. I can't think why on earth it would work here in Australia.'

Perhaps Slim Dusty was right about a pub with no beer. But still, Paddy humours me and refers the question to his chief executive, Brian Kearney, and I wait, hoping there's a hidden network of non-drinking publicans poised to open Melbourne's first alcohol-free bars and offer a smorgasbord of interesting soft drinks to see me through the rest of the year. When the response comes back, in an emailed statement, I'm disappointed. 'Hospitality businesses respond to customer demand and this is prevalent in the hotel industry where a wide range of non-alcohol drinks are also available for customers.' We may have to agree to disagree on that one.

Still, at least a night-time diet of soft drinks is saving me money. According to the Australian Bureau of Statistics, the average Aussie spends $31 a week on booze. That's the equivalent of about eight full-strength pots of beer. Interestingly, people of my vintage, Generation X, spent slightly more per week ($33) than Generation Y ($30). I'm not sure who they surveyed, but it certainly wasn't anyone I know. After some back-of-the-envelope calculations, I'd say that, at a conservative estimate, my spending on alcohol was about three times that amount. I'd usually buy at least one $20 to $25 bottle of wine a week, to bring either to a restaurant or to a friend's house for dinner. If I went out one night on the weekend, I'd usually have six or seven drinks (probably more if it was a late night). I prefer bottled beer over tap beer, so that's about $7 a drink. Then there's the taxi home, which usually costs about $25. All up, that's about $100 a week on booze. If I went out two nights over the weekend, which I often did, I could almost double that amount. That places my annual spending on alcohol at somewhere around $10,000. In 20 years, I may have spent $200,000 on booze — that's almost somebody's mortgage. A sobering thought indeed.

I discuss this with Chris Raine, who's in town for the Australian Drug Foundation's International Conference on Drugs and Young People, where he's giving a presentation about *Hello Sunday Morning*. He saved a whopping $12,000 during his year off the booze. Catching up with him is like getting a glimpse into my future: he's one of the few people I know who's been sober longer than I have. He seems to have survived. In fact, he's thriving. At the conference, he begins by trying to persuade the Melbourne Convention Centre audience to have a crack at a three-month non-drinking challenge, and there are few takers. Then he tells them about the freak-themed costume party he went to during his year without alcohol. Dressed in a gimp mask, a superhero cape, red undies, and not much else, he turned up completely sober and had what he describes as one of the most emotionally revealing moments of his life. He realised that if he could do that without alcohol, he could do anything. The red undies came to symbolise all that *HSM* offers: bravery, confidence, fun, and inspiration. Drinking water when everyone around you is knocking back beers is like wearing your undies on the outside — you're exposed, vulnerable, and different. It forces you to be fearless. Chris tells the room that there are now 700 people around Australia embracing the *HSM* challenge. Watching him speak, I'm overcome with a sense of pride and purpose. This is how you change a culture: one person at a time.

LIFE HAS A perverse way of kicking you in the teeth when things are going well. When I bounce into work today, it is waiting there, like a bomb, in my inbox: an email from Fairfax management. Our subeditors are being made redundant. Their work will be outsourced, effective almost immediately. About 90 staff from *The Age* and *The Sydney Morning Herald* will lose their jobs. Shock and disbelief ripple through the office, as more people turn on their computers and discover this nasty surprise.

A meeting of the *Age* house committee — a delegation of journalists, including me, who work with the union to protect jobs, entitlements, and the quality of our newspapers — is called. We're all stunned. Redundancies are never pretty. There will be shock, grief, and anger. But these job losses represent a bigger truth: newspapers are dying. How many more cuts can we endure before there's no blood left to spill? We worry that getting rid of our subeditors — guardians of the quality, accuracy, and integrity that have been the hallmarks of these proud papers for nearly 160 years — will be like removing the foundations of the building. How long before it comes crumbling down around us?

As the day goes on, disbelief turns to fury. There's talk of a strike. Reporters feel powerless, and want to show their support for the subs. During the last round of redundancies, in 2008, editorial staff walked off the job and went straight to the pub — where else would you go to show your solidarity? We drank and hugged, and raised a cheer when our strike action appeared as one of the lead items on the ABC evening news. It was a four-day strike, and I drank a lot during it: to relieve stress, to bond with workmates, and to obscure the obvious. I wonder how I'm going to get through this without alcohol.

The announcement makes me fear for the future. Apart from bar work, the newspaper game is the only career I've ever known. It's what I've wanted to do since I was a ten-year-old, producing newspapers and magazines with craft paper and glue on my parents' kitchen table. But my job, at least for now, is safe. Unlike some of my colleagues, I'm not facing unemployment or contemplating selling my home. In light of that, drowning my sorrows in booze seems a little self-indulgent. It doesn't stop the urge to reach for the bottle, though.

When I get home that night, I'm desperately craving a drink — a pull-the-cork-out-with-my-teeth, neck-the-bottle, and-belt-out-love-songs kind of craving. I'm so tense my shoulders are up somewhere around my earlobes, and my jaw is clamped so tightly my teeth hurt. The three unopened bottles of red wine on my kitchen benchtop are so hard to ignore, they might as well be doing the can-can and cheering my name with pom poms. I can see myself taking that first sip. I can feel the muscles uncoiling, and the jangled nerves settling down. It might only take one glass to get peace.

But somehow I manage to close my ears to alcohol's siren song. Eventually, my breathing returns to a normal rhythm and my heart stops fluttering. I'm stronger than I thought.

As the week drags on, it gets harder. The days are long. We spend hours in emotionally charged union meetings, trying to figure out ways to save even one job. It punches a hole in my guts and leaves me exhausted. The stop-work staff meetings are the worst. The house committee has to try to persuade the editorial floor not to walk —

as much as we all want to make a public display of our strength and unity, we don't think this is the way to do it. Instead, we try to convince our colleagues that a high-profile public campaign, highlighting how the outsourcing threatens the very future of our mastheads, is the way to go. It's a strategy that many staff members oppose. There is anger; there are tears and recriminations. It's awful. For the subs, it must be agonising. Staff are crying and hugging one another in stairwells, as if a nuclear holocaust is coming. Beneath our emotion is the grim knowledge that there's probably nothing we can do. What we love is in its death throes; it feels like we're fighting for a mercy killing.

It's hard not to succumb to a drink at the end of the day. It's really fucking hard. There are times this week when I would gladly raffle off a vital organ for one sip of beer. One evening, being around a friend as she blithely chugs back a Peroni is so teeth-grindingly excruciating that I have to use all my powers of restraint not to karate-kick the stubby from her hand and run wailing into the night, to the nearest bottle shop.

As I struggle not to cave in, I realise how much I've relied on alcohol to calm my brain after a tough day at work. It gave me a reprieve from the racing thoughts, from the doubts and fears. Not only did it soothe the anxiety, but it also allowed me to paper over my shortcomings. Without it, I'm being forced to face my biggest flaws. Sometimes I lash out without thinking. I can be negative and controlling. And I can't blame the hangover; I can't blame the beer. This is me. It's uncomfortable, but staring my weaknesses squarely in the eye is the only way to foster change. I will persevere and prevail.

In fact, alcohol has been my quick-fix medication whenever life serves up a shit sandwich. Six years ago, when I found out that my grandmother had died, I left the pub I was working in and took a bottle of vodka home with me to numb the pain. It seemed the acceptable reaction to grief. When my parents announced that they were getting a divorce, I called my ex-boyfriend and we went straight to a bar. It didn't end well.

But alcohol is a depressant. When I drink too much booze, it feels as if I am driving a bulldozer through my nervous system. It depletes levels of the 'happy chemical', serotonin, in my brain, and raises my heart rate. The morning after, as my body tries to fight the sedative effects of a bucketload of beer, it can lead to a heightened sense of hyperactivity. Alcohol might 'take the edge off', but the next morning those edges are sharper and cut deeper. Yet I'm not alone: the post-work glass of wine is a nationally accepted way to unwind. Earlier this year, when Australians were questioned as part of a federal government survey on national wellbeing, 40 per cent admitted to using alcohol to cope with stress. Only half found it an effective strategy. But our knowledge that it's not helpful doesn't stop us from relying on it — alcohol is still the default remedy in times of crisis. A stiff drink is the panacea for shock. I remember watching news footage of Queenslanders who had lost everything in 2010's devastating floods. As they waded through the remnants of their lives, some of them told journos, 'What can you do but have a beer?'

At work, the mood is bleak. Despite all of our strategising and negotiating, and a public campaign that garners the support of dozens of Australia's most prominent leaders and thinkers — including former prime minister Malcolm Fraser, singer-songwriter Paul Kelly, writers Peter Carey and John Pilger, and an array of former state premiers and Australians of the year — there's no sign that management will back down on the redundancies. No-one's saying it, but there's a palpable sense of inevitability to it all. The unspoken fear is that someday, and that day may be soon, newspapers will no longer be printed. We're ready to embrace the digital revolution and to accept a degree of rationalisation if it will help us to survive, but what will survival cost? What will become of our craft when the last of these skilled practitioners, with newspaper ink pulsing through their veins, are put out to pasture? When they walk out the door for the last time, it won't just be friends, colleagues, and decades of experience that we'll lose. The door will close on tradition.

As I brace for possible industrial action, and for the days of hard drinking in which I can't participate, I start to think about the role that alcohol has in that tradition. Journalism is a recipe for heavy drinking: the long hours, the late deadlines, and the often extraordinary events we witness. The comradeship between subs and reporters, working together to get a late-breaking story into the paper, was traditionally cemented over beers when the presses started rolling. It was no surprise to me when I learned that it was journalists at the *Bulletin* magazine who led the push against Australia's temperance movement, fighting any moves to restrict the sale of alcohol. Boozing is a journalistic institution.

In my tabloid days in Scotland, retiring to the pub when your shift was over was an almost daily occurrence. Here, ten years later, it's not so common — although there are some notable exceptions. In particular, there was the infamous 12-hour farewell lunch that a group of *Sunday Age* staff organised for our colleague Cam, who was off to spend a year in New York. What started out as a civilised pub lunch on a Tuesday afternoon ended up as a marathon drinking session. We sat down to eat at noon, and left when the pub shut its doors at midnight. And older journos talk fondly of *The Age*'s Bog Bar, which convened after the first edition, in a locker room off the men's toilets. Both sexes were welcome, but membership was required.

Bonding over beers in the pub with workmates is more than just a social gathering or a chance to get plastered. It can be a way to process the trauma on which we regularly report. It also offers schooling for younger journalists, providing a convivial environment in which to learn from veteran reporters who have covered wars, disasters, world cups, and Olympics. In years past, a reporter repeatedly turning in sloppy copy might get some quiet advice from a subeditor in the pub, but now we're losing the chance for some of that interaction. Soon, the people editing our stories won't even be in the same building.

To better understand the historical role that drinking has played in journalism, I talk to some of *The Age*'s longest-serving reporters. I catch up with Steve Butcher — or Butch, as he's known in the newsroom. He's our award-winning chief court reporter. He's also an old-school, pavement-pounding grafter, who started his career in 1972 at Melbourne's notorious *Truth* newspaper, a Rupert Murdoch–owned publication, which he sums up as a renegade outfit offering 'screaming headlines, breasts, sport, and brothel ads'. Heavy drinking was the predominant pastime at *Truth*. 'You met contacts in the pub; you met police in the pub; lawyers, judges in the pub; crooks in the pub. If you didn't drink, you weren't trusted. So if you wanted a yarn, for people to absolutely open up, they're a lot more comfortable when they're off the bench, out of the police station, away from chambers, and they get a few beers in them. There's a famous saying that a drunk man says what a sober man thinks. Loose lips provide stories.'

Butch says that the art of 'becoming a chameleon' — blending into your contacts' environment — is the key to establishing rapport and earning trust. If that means sitting in the park and eating a sandwich, he'll do that. If the contact wants to grab a coffee or go for a walk, he'll oblige them. But more secrets are spilled over a few beers.

Oiling up sources over a liquid lunch used to be a management-sanctioned practice. Reporters were given free rein to rack up large expense bills in the pub, as long as the sessions spawned the occasional ripping yarn. 'We'd have huge nights at the boozer, where you'd turn up to work the next day with a shocking hangover, and by about 11 o'clock someone would say, "Feel like a beer?" "Aw, yeah."

You were thinking, it's going to kill me, but you got over there and before you knew it, you were pissed again. It was fantastic,' he says, with a wide grin.

These days, expenses are more tightly monitored. Set limits on 'meal' allowances have made boozy afternoons with sources an alien concept for many young reporters. Butch believes that the new generation of journalists are losing the 'getting your boots dirty' skill of building contacts; we're all far more office-bound, and isolated behind our computer screens, than ever before. 'More than half of this office I'd transplant back there if I could, for 18 months at *Truth* — the drinking and carrying on and working hard and being screamed at. They would be a lot more sharp-edged than they are. Everyone's so fit and healthy these days. Nowadays you take people for a coffee, which is boring unless you're going to put a whisky in it. There's no doubt some of them [young journalists] are missing that opportunity to get out on the booze and have a drink with a couple of lawyers or coppers. At Christmas, every police station had a party, and the clerks of court would have Christmas parties and prosecutors would have barbecues, and the drunkenness and the outrageousness was just fantastic. You'd take booze and get blind, and fights would start, but it was all in.' These days, he adds mournfully, media companies are more interested in 'arse protection'.

Butch's good mate John 'Sly' Silvester, *The Age*'s veteran crime reporter and co-author of the *Underbelly* books, believes that newspaper journalism's historical association with heavy drinking is less to do with alcohol being a lubricant and more to do with the long, unsociable hours that came from late deadlines. 'All of these professions that were the last to break that strong alcohol dominance were almost all shift workers, all high-pressure jobs, many of them life-and-death jobs. So the coppers, barristers who worked long hours and worked in very strange environments together; the journos; the nurses, doctors in casualty — you shared your problems together.

Today, we've got counsellors; we've got different ways of dealing with stuff. In the old days, the sort of rule was: go and get pissed, talk your problems out, front up tomorrow, have a shower and a shave, and off we go.'

Drinking was common among reporters and subs working night shifts in the 1970s and 1980s, due to a combination of 'comradeship, loneliness, and boredom' as they waited for the big story to break. 'You'd slip over to the pub because you'd done the crossword. There was no internet — this is 8.30 at night and you're working to 11 — so you may as well go and have a few beers as just sit there. No subs went home before the first edition, so everyone was there at midnight. There was nothing for them to do except go home to an empty house. They'd spread the newspapers out, open the fridge, and get some beers out. When I started, the police club was one of the few places you could get packaged grog after ten o'clock at night, so on occasions we'd have the editor ring and say, "We've run out of booze. Can you get us some slabs?"'

Drinking on the job was so accepted Sly remembers reporters turning up to work pissed, and management complaining about the number of empty beer cans in the police-rounds car. Drink-driving was a regular and unremarkable occurrence. The close social bond between journos and police officers meant that crime reporters were often green-lighted. Earlier deadlines, fewer editions, the demise of evening newspapers, and the introduction of drink-driving laws have helped change that drinking culture, which Sly says is not a bad thing — for journos or police. 'When you talk about the police culture, about working a million hours and then going down the police club and just sleeping on a desk, and then doing a raid, it sounds good. But look at the number of them who died when they hit poles, died in car accidents. Or there were police raids with cops who were over .05 — there were occasions when it was just a miracle people didn't get shot.

'There were night-shift barbecues, where the patrol cars would pull up, have a barbecue, and then drive up and down the freeway to get their clicks up so it looked like they'd been working. But then, one day, there was a fatal accident involving a divvy van going through a red light after they'd been to a barbecue. They weren't drunk — they weren't even .05 — but that was the end of that. While it was fun to be there, it mightn't have been fun if I was at home and I'd just been burgled and the coppers weren't turning up because they were having sausages on the Yarra.'

But while heavy drinking was rife among law and justice reporters and their circles, both Butch and Sly tell me that it was nothing compared to the shenanigans that used to go on in the Canberra press gallery. Working in a rabbit warren of tiny offices, shrouded in a fug of cigarette smoke, political reporters lived a life of over-indulgence, hundreds of kilometres away from their newspaper's headquarters and the scrutiny of their editors. One of the original party animals was Tony Wright, who has racked up nearly 25 years in the press gallery, starting at *The Canberra Times* in 1987. He now works for *The Age* as national editor, dividing his time between Melbourne and the nation's capital. When we catch up, he looks back on his journalistic career, which began in 1970, and tells me that hard drinking was endemic throughout that decade, and remained so through the 1980s and well into the 1990s.

He has a theory about the drinking and loutish behaviour. The hard-nosed journos, predominantly men, were overcompensating for the fact that they spent their days in offices typing, which was traditionally considered women's work. They were the 'Wild West of the clerical class', he says. 'The editor would say, "We're off to the pub for a counter meal," you'd knock back seven or eight schooners, and then you'd come back and fall asleep on your typewriter. That was just what you did. It was the social glue.'

But the wild lifestyle took its toll on many mates. There were more than a few hard drinkers who ended up unable to function. Some went on to develop alcoholic dementia. 'A lot of the so-called legendary journos made their names among their peers just as much for their behaviour at the bar, or for their ability to hold alcohol or still file with one hand over their eyes. But back then nobody thought of it as "problems with alcohol". It just meant they could drink more than anybody else, or that they were wilder. But yeah, marriages fell apart, lives fell apart.'

Sly had told me something similar. The war stories from the halcyon days don't tell the whole tale. 'More often than not, if you drill down to the end of the story, the person died prematurely or became very lonely. There was a series of working alcoholics. There were people who lost their way in that culture.'

Sly believes that the hard-drinking reputation of crime reporters, and the police officers they befriended, was part of a myth constructed to help maintain the boys'-club mentality in a politically incorrect era. It was the kind of macho culture that, in the late 1970s, saw one female reporter sent home from work for wearing trousers. 'It was that idea that girlies couldn't possibly look at a dead body. You can't have a girl go down the pub and drink ten pots. Of course, some of the best crime reporters in the world have been female.'

When feminism took hold, many female reporters embraced the drinking culture as a way of being taken seriously in a man's world. In Canberra, journalists and politicians would mingle at the non-members bar in Old Parliament House, or have long lunches together at the National Press Club or a handful of favoured restaurants. Boozy Friday sessions became so sacrosanct that a tacit agreement was reached between journalists and politicians: on Friday afternoons, no press conferences would be held, nor media releases issued. Things often got out of hand in these drinking sessions. In an incident still talked about today, two of Australia's oldest and most venerated political reporters charged at each other 'like a pair of old bulls' during a heated argument in the Press Club bar, their bellies bouncing off each other upon impact. 'This was accepted behaviour,' Tony says.

Graphix, an upstairs late-night bar in Kingston, was also a popular haunt with pollies and journos, particularly on budget night. It didn't start jumping till after 2.00 a.m. 'Blood was spilled, scores were settled, and marriages went upside down,' said Tony. But he remembers it most for being the venue where, in the late 1980s, he and some colleagues invented the sport of 'ottering'. 'One night, a few of us worked out that if we put our hands behind our backs and stood at the top of the stairs and fell forward, you would slide on your bellies flat to the boards and get to the bottom. And if you had your head up, you wouldn't get too much carpet rash. Politicians would actually come along to watch it because a lot of people in the press gallery got into it. It made planking look pretty bloody ordinary.'

But it was a perilous pursuit. On the same night that an ABC television reporter fractured her wrist while attempting the advanced 'double otter' with a colleague, a *Sydney Morning Herald* photographer broke his leg in a solo feat. Their efforts made such an impact on the then federal treasurer, Peter Costello, that he shared them with the nation during a live National Press Club speech following the delivery of his 1998 budget.

Hazardous drinking games aside, the relationships formed under the influence of alcohol had professional benefits for both politicians and reporters. Tony says that secrets were passed to inebriated journalists prior to Paul Keating's leadership challenge on Bob Hawke. 'Keating's people made sure that journalists were extremely well briefed at Graphix, very late at night, about what Keating was up to and what a dreadful bastard Hawke was. That was all because of lubrication. Notes would be taken in the toilets and so forth. Somebody confided one night that Peter Walsh, who was the finance minister, had named Hawke "Old Jellyback". Suddenly it started appearing in newspapers. A lot of unsourced stories from that period came out of those drinking holes very, very late at night, quite often with the sun glinting off Lake Burley Griffin when you were driving home.'

I know, from speaking to friends and colleagues in the Canberra press gallery, that drinking has not gone out of fashion in the nation's capital. Journalists still mix with politicians, and budget night remains one of the booziest events in the political calendar. But there's no doubt that things have changed. Thirty years ago, newspapers provided their senior political reporters with large houses, where lavish parties would be thrown and journalists, diplomats, public servants, and politicians would get drunk together. The perks are gone these days, and there are few 'lifers' left. Reporters might spend a year or two as a Canberra correspondent, using it as a stepping stone before returning to a more senior role at head office. The chummy relationship between reporters and parliamentarians has changed, too — politicians are more closely media-managed than ever before.

For Tony, it was Paul Keating's decision to privatise the catering at Parliament House that sparked the beginning of the end of the entente cordiale. The new contractors deemed the non-members bar unprofitable, closing it down. It was later turned into an aerobics centre. 'It changed a lot of things because suddenly there was no central social outlet where politicians and staffers and journos could gather in a totally informal way, pass secrets back and forth, and drink a lot and get a bit indiscreet. Things moved out of Parliament House, and a couple of other restaurants around the place became meeting places, but they were much more formal and much more open, and people could see who was talking to whom. The new Parliament House also allowed politicians to disappear into their big offices, protected by receptionists, so it really grew apart, the political class from the journalist class.'

The Prime Minister still holds annual Christmas drinks at the Lodge for the media, but Tony says they're sedate, stage-managed affairs. Not like the parties thrown by Bob Hawke, who, although he didn't drink for the 12 years he was in parliament, would invite his favourite journos upstairs to play pool and drink till dawn. John Howard's shindigs were also a high point for Tony. 'One year, I was stumbling around and I went over to get a drink, but the waiter said, "Sorry, the drinks are off now. It's over. Mr Howard says the drinks go off at this time." So I went back and said, "John, this is fucking outrageous — you've turned the taps off." He said, "What are you talking about, Tony? I know nothing about that." And I said, "Well, you better go and talk to your caterers, because we've just been told we can't have any more drinks." So off he went to talk to them, and next minute the grog's back on, and everyone's yahooing and carrying on. Then I said, "There's a lot of young journos here who have never seen the Lodge" — because they have a big marquee out the back for the party — "I think you should do a guided tour." He said, "Well, Tony, that's a good idea." So off we go, and we started this conga line weaving through the Lodge and carrying on, and we ended up at the grand piano playing Christmas tunes and singing off-key, and it went on quite late into the night.'

At another of Howard's Christmas parties, a well-known press-gallery photographer stripped down to his jocks and jumped into the pool. Howard was amused; his wife, Janette, wasn't. At the following year's party, there was a cover stretched over the pool.

As Tony points out, it's hard to imagine Julia Gillard or Tony Abbott playing host to such high jinks without it turning into a controversy. For reporters, the demands of the 24-hour news cycle, and of increasingly discerning media consumers who expect stories to be packaged with interactive graphics, pictures, and video, leave little time for long sessions in the pub.

But it doesn't stop me from feeling like I'm letting the team down by not joining in. Clearly, journalists are big drinkers — it's just who we are and who we've always been. I'm betraying the traditions of my profession by opting out.

Tony disagrees. 'I don't think it's so exclusive to journalism as people imagine, this drinking culture, because you'd go to other trades and alcohol was … alcohol was Australia.'

He may be right. When I first met Chris Raine in 2010, it was a few days after the Quills, the Melbourne Press Club's annual awards for Victorian journalism — a night notorious as the biggest media piss-up of the year. As we were having coffee in the *Age* cafe, Butch walked past. We swapped stories about the wild night we'd had, and which journo had disgraced themselves the most. I recounted how I was so drunk at the afterparty that I tottered over on my red satin stilettos and took a tumble ankle-deep into a fish pond. We laughed, and as Butch walked off I pointed out to Chris that this was exactly why I couldn't accept his challenge of three months without alcohol. 'It's too hard in this culture,' I said. 'Journalists are such big drinkers.' He smiled knowingly. He'd heard it before. Lawyers, nurses, advertising executives, tradesmen, flight attendants, architects — they all insist that their industry has a reputation for hard drinking.

In the end, I don't have to worry about surviving a strike sober. We avoid industrial action and have a huge public rally instead. It's heartening to see so many Melburnians turn out to support the newspaper that has such cultural significance to their city. We manage to hang on to some of our subs, but many of them go. The farewells are heart-wrenching. And at every leaving do organised by management, no soft drinks are offered. Our professional stereotype prevails.

June

I BUMP INTO my editor at the traffic lights outside the *Age* building, on the way to work. She has something to tell me, and apparently it can't wait. 'I was thinking last night about your situation. Maybe you're one of those people who should just never drink.'

I'm a bit taken aback — but there's more. 'You know, there are some people who can't drink because they don't know when to stop. I'm not saying that's you, but maybe if you can't drink moderately, you just shouldn't drink at all.'

Given that she encouraged all of her staff to sign up for a month off the booze for Febfast and lasted three days before succumbing to a post-work glass of wine, I feel this is a tad rich. But the underlying message stays with me. First Kerri-Anne, now my editor: people think that I have a drinking problem. Yet would an alcoholic just be able to stop? Would they hit a wall of stress and get around it without opening a bottle? Nevertheless, it gets me pondering the nature of addiction. How many people slide from binge drinking to all-out dependency? Is it an easy transition?

To explore this further, I arrange to meet one of my favourite contacts. Professor Jon Currie is the head of addiction medicine at Melbourne's St Vincent's Hospital. He was also the chair of the

National Health and Medical Research Council committee that revised Australia's alcohol guidelines in 2009 — the committee that, after exhaustive scientific review, concluded that if we want to reduce our lifetime risk of disease, accident, and injury, we should have, on average, no more than two standard drinks a day, and no more than four in any one sitting. Jon, who now only drinks according to these guidelines, insists that consuming any more will sharply increase the risk of ill health.

We meet in the hospital cafeteria. When he arrives late because his previous appointment ran over time, he's flustered and full of apologies. But I don't mind; over my years of covering the health beat, he's been enormously helpful, and always generous with his time. I tell him about my year without booze, and ask about alcohol dependency — and whether a regular binge drinker who loves to party can end up with a full-blown drinking problem. He tells me that addiction is a complex risk-equation: exposure plus genetics plus environment. It means that if you have a family history of dependency and move in circles where heavy drinking or drug use is rife, you could be in trouble; between 6 and 10 per cent of the population falls into that category. And while your socioeconomic status may play a part in your access to treatment, addiction is not a respecter of social class. 'You can get as dependent on champagne or good red wine as you can on Jim Beam,' he says, telling me that many of his patients are young professionals.

From what he sees in terms of numbers walking through the doors at St Vincent's, it seems that there are far more people in trouble than ever before. And they're getting younger: Jon says many addiction clinics are starting to treat children aged 13 or 14 (the youngest child he's seen was ten). Their drug of choice is almost always alcohol. 'It's very small compared with the adult population, but our worry is that what we used to see at 25, in terms of patients with alcohol problems, we're now seeing at 18 to 20. Kids in their last three years of high school are particularly worrying. The levels of drinking at that 15-, 16-year-old age are really quite a worry in schools now, and it seems to be escalating.'

I try to imagine a ten-year-old alcoholic. My niece is nearly seven. The idea that in just over three years she could be chugging back bottles of Scotch is impossible to imagine. I wonder if he's trying to scare me. Is it really possible that a child could be ruined by booze by their tenth birthday? Perhaps sensing my scepticism, he tells me a story that eliminates any doubt. 'We just admitted someone the other day who was wheelchair-bound at 24 from brain damage. Couldn't walk because the balance centres in the brain had been hit by alcohol, like a massive stroke. That's not a day or two of alcohol, that's probably ten-plus years. You extrapolate back and ask yourself, how the hell could this happen at 24? Well, he must have been drinking at 15, 16? No. He was drinking at ten. These consequences: you'll start to see them not at 35 but at 25, and you'll get this slow shift to younger ages of what are really chronic diseases — liver disease, cancer, brain damage; it will start to happen earlier and earlier. Young people are drinking earlier, and the proportion that is drinking heavily is climbing. We're going to reap the harvest of that in a period of five or ten years.'

He refers to a Victorian survey released last year that showed 42 per cent of 16- to 24-year-olds had drunk more than 20 drinks — almost three bottles of wine — in one sitting at least once a year. That's a massive night, even by my standards. More than half of them experienced blackouts: they got so pissed that they couldn't remember what happened. It's the stuff of parents' nightmares. But not every binge drinker will end up with a brain so saturated with vodka that they're confined to a wheelchair. What is it that turns a weekend party-animal into an addict?

'You must have had this situation where everyone goes out and has a good time, but for the rest of the week no-one does it — except one friend, who then finds the next party, and the next party, and the next party. They're the ones who end up really sick, and rapidly moving along that pathway,' he tells me. 'That's the most susceptible group, and the most difficult to treat because we really have to keep them and alcohol separate; they just can't really be exposed. For that group, even after a year of not using it, they are still likely to go back and become re-addicted. Even a year later, the brain is likely to be primed to want to go back to it.'

I'm suspicious as to why he mentions a year. Does he think that my brain is primed, and raring to go back to booze? I ask him how easy it is to move along the addiction pathway; he tells me that it's easier than most people realise. It's a subtle creep. The number of drinks in each binge steadily rises, and the gap between sessions gets smaller. At this point, mornings-after are no longer hangovers but mini-withdrawals, as the body and mind begin to crave more booze. Thousands of young Australians are drinking in this way, he says, largely on Thursday-, Friday-, and Saturday-night heavy sessions. Come Monday and Tuesday, they find it hard to function.

'Essentially, what you're looking at is brain toxicity two or three days past the episode. This is really quite frightening in terms of economic performance for the country because how many people are out there accident-prone or not working as well because they've got this problem on Monday or Tuesday? Part of it is sleep and part of it is withdrawal — brain-chemical changes that have happened with the heavy intake. Young people are much more tolerant of the physical effects of alcohol, so they can drink more without becoming as intoxicated, and they don't get the warning signs of four drinks, six drinks, eight drinks. But their brains are much more susceptible to damage because they're still developing. The risk is that young people who binge drink will have impairment of subtle cognitive function as they grow older. If you expose the brain early, there's also the risk of the increased incidence of mental-health issues, particularly anxiety and depression, and an increased risk of drug and alcohol dependence later in life.'

I think of my own struggles with anxiety and depression, and, for the first time, consider whether they were exacerbated or even caused by my early binge-drinking habits. At 14 and 15, my friends and I would pair up and share bottles of Martini Bianco undiluted (we thought it was supposed to be drunk like wine) before heading out with our fake IDs to drink vodka and Coke in pubs. We'd often vomit; occasionally, one of us would pass out. We've all grown up to be healthy, and to have successful jobs and relationships. We're not like the brain-damaged alcoholics whom I've written about in *The Age*. But what Jon's suggesting is that my brain may have been changing in ways that I didn't even realise.

'We're not talking about people dragging their knuckles and dribbling into their Wheaties. We're talking about subtle impairments, which means that you're at 95 when you could have been at 100 per cent,' he says. 'Given how much effort so many mums put into ensuring what's best for their babies, it's just extraordinary that they'll have the kids drinking when all this work's gone into getting tutors and doing everything they can to optimise their chances at VCE or HSC. It's this misguided business of it being better to introduce them to alcohol in the family environment — there's not a lot of evidence that that works, and there's a reasonable amount of evidence that in fact it can be quite dangerous.'

But if heavy drinking as a teenager could set you up for problems later in life, what damage are you doing if you're still drinking that way at 35? 'The issues of adolescence are about development, but at 35 it's about function. If you already have a predisposition to depression and anxiety, that can be significantly exacerbated by drinking. Conversely, if you do lots of drinking, you can precipitate depression even if you're not particularly that way inclined. In terms of waking up the next morning, it seems fairly clear that older people do not tolerate heavy drinking sessions as well.'

In the last couple of years, my hangovers had become increasingly mind-numbing; I'd often find myself at work on Monday or Tuesday morning with a brain that felt like half a kilogram of mince. On some level, I guess I knew that mince-brain wasn't a sign of optimal health, but there's something about hearing the words 'brain toxicity' that leaves me cold. What has 20 years of drinking done to my wiring? I have joked about my head being a brain-cell graveyard, but I didn't seriously believe that I was inflicting lasting damage. In fact, as galactically stupid as it sounds, particularly for a health reporter, I've never really thought of alcohol as a drug. I'm reminded of my teetotaller friend Nick, who describes getting pissed as a delicate balancing act between drinking just enough poison to give you a buzz, but not enough to kill you. 'For all the wine-tasting and brandy snifters and expensive cellars, it's essentially no different from sniffing petrol or chroming. It's just dressed up,' he said. 'Can you imagine businessmen with plastic bags spraying paint and saying, "Why, yes, it's a 1954 Dulux. Yes, that was a good year. Is that the enamel? Ah, lovely."'

As I mull over the potentially changed chemistry of my brain, Jon begins to ask questions about my habits. He wants to know if I've found myself drinking more in each 'episode', as the years have passed. My ability to hold my liquor and be the last one standing has always been a source of pride; I thought it made me hardcore. I am Scottish, after all. He shakes his head and tells me it means that my tolerance has become so high through years of heavy drinking that I need to consume more to get the same effect of being drunk. I don't like where this is going. I came here to talk about the patients who visit his addiction clinic, not to discuss my nights out. But it seems that through his eyes, in some ways, he can't separate us. It dawns on me: he's taking a clinical history.

'Have you ever blacked out through drinking?' he asks. I think back to Melbourne Cup Day last year — a barbecue at a friend's place that started at lunchtime and ended around 10.00 p.m. It was a laugh. Hats were compulsory: there was a chicken hat, a pig hat, a couple of trilbies, a straw boater, and one Saddam Hussein mask. I chose a See You Jimmy tartan bonnet with Viking horns. I drank champers, which is not my usual tipple, and by mid-afternoon I was hammered. The champagne is surely the only explanation for why I have very few memories of events after about 5.00 p.m., including of how I got home. Honestly, it wasn't the first time — I had a couple of those nights last year.

'We know that multiple episodes of blackout is a significant risk of brain impairment, not to mention the risk of what happens when you're blacked out,' Jon tells me, with a look to suggest that only dumb luck has saved me from more serious consequences. 'That sort of effect on the brain becomes worrying in a 35-year-old. One of the most interesting things about drinkers in the 30-to-40 age group is what has happened to their cognitive function: they often have the cognitive processes of a 60-year-old when they're only 40. They're tired in the afternoon, they don't have the memory they used to have, and they can't multi-process.'

The tips of my fingers are tingling. My mouth is suddenly dry. I have often felt like a geriatric when I'm struggling to string sentences together on a Monday morning. My short-term memory is woeful. When I ask him if he was shocked when he read about my binge-drinking double life, he doesn't sugar-coat his answer. 'I'm not surprised that a health reporter would drink that much because the definition of addiction is the compulsive seeking out and using of the drug even knowing the negative health consequences. There's a total cognitive dissonance between what I do and what I know. You can know it all, but it doesn't stop you wanting it.'

Hold up. The definition of what?

'Those levels [of drinking] and those effects you were experiencing, that's representative of subtle or mild pathology. You don't need to be Sherlock Holmes to see that it must have been taking a chunk out of your brain performance, and that's a worry because you want that performance at 60 or 80 — and if there's already impairment at the age of 35, what's going to happen in another ten years? That has a suggestion of incipient dependence. It's slightly pre-malignant addiction. Like pre-malignant cancer; it's cells that are not quite healthy. This isn't, "Oh gosh, she's an alcoholic," but, "Gee, there are aspects there which are more than we would expect with somebody who hasn't got any issue at all with it."'

There are certain phrases in life that you hope never to hear but will be forever seared into your memory, such as 'Collingwood premiership' or 'geriatric sex aid' or 'pre-malignant addiction'. In that moment, my year without alcohol becomes more than just an interesting social experiment. What I have considered normal for years has a medical term. Like pre-cancerous cells that may grow to create tissue-destroying disease, my nights on the piss could be the precursors to alcoholism. If I already show signs of 'incipient dependence', how many more beers will it take to reach my tipping point? Perhaps my editor was right: maybe I should never drink.

But I can't help wondering, is this doctor simply out of touch? A lot of my friends drink like this. I'm not even the biggest drinker in the group. Nobody can be expected to have no more than two standard drinks a day — that would be a very short night in the pub. The way I drink is normal.

'There's a difference between normal and healthy,' Jon says, in a statement so profound that it seems to echo back at me in surround sound. 'We have to ask ourselves if we are going to get, over time, a gradual increase in this being acceptable, and are we risking pickling the brains of future generations because we are setting them up with an environment where this kind of excessive drinking is more and more normal?'

I feel as if I've just been told the world is flat. I knew that I was drinking more than was healthy; I don't have to be chugging wine for breakfast to know that alcohol has a hold on me. When I tell him about my heroin-like chocolate habit, he says that this might also be indicative of an addictive predisposition. Suddenly, my treatment on *Kerri-Anne* seems a little less outrageous than I thought.

I don't want him to see how freaked out I am. Adopting an air of casual curiosity — slightly betrayed by the shrillness of my voice — I ask him what he thinks will happen if I go back to drinking at the end of the year. He describes the situation as being like an elastic band stretched out to its maximum point of tension. Eventually, it will prove too much, and the band will snap back. He suggests that I might want to try something called 'controlled drinking', which he uses with patients who are not full-blown alcoholics but have dependency problems and need help to improve their drinking habits. Prior to going out, you nominate how much you plan to drink — preferably no more than four standard drinks, in accordance with the national guidelines — and stick to that. This is the template you always use. If, over a period of time, you find you're failing to stick to it, then it might be time to consider not drinking at all.

But if it were that easy, we'd all be sticking to the national guidelines. How many times have I heard friends say, 'I'm not having a big night,' only to find that a couple of beers has turned into a 3.00 a.m. bender? Controlled drinking has one fundamental flaw — every beer chips away at the powers of reasoning and self-control you need to help you make good decisions. I find that once I have a taste for it, alcohol only gets more appealing as the night goes on. Perhaps abstinence is an easier choice.

Jon offers to conduct some tests: brain scans and neuro-psychological tests that may reveal whether two decades of binge drinking have damaged my brain's structure and function. He tells me that researchers now know the brain doesn't stop developing until well into our twenties, not in the late teens, as previously thought. Binge drinking from a young age may have had an impact on my neurocognitive development — particularly on the brain structures that transport the chemical serotonin, which regulates mood and memory. I'm curious about his offer, but also scared. I've sensed for some time that my brain is not working to its full potential, especially during those protracted hangovers. My memory is really bad, and my moods have been erratic from an early age, but I'd always presumed that was just my personality. Maybe some truths are best left unspoken.

At the end of my chat with Jon, I'm not sure whether to thank him for the interview or hand over my Medicare card. He tells me that if I do go back to drinking, I should be careful. My tolerance will be at an all-time low. One beer could be enough to get me drunk. Oh well, at least I'll be a cheap date, I joke. But as I walk back to my car, I'm not laughing. It's dark already, and the evening air bites. I hug my notepad to my chest, keeping the details of my intervention close to my heart.

I'M GOING HOME to Scotland to see my family. I miss them all dreadfully, and often wish that circumstances had taken me to a life in a city slightly closer to Edinburgh and the people I love the most. Trips home are always emotionally charged, but this time there will be an added element of self-discovery: by going home, I hope to retrace my drinking steps.

Scotland was where I first experienced the seductive embrace of alcohol. I have displayed my drinking dexterity with great patriotism, seeing it as a sign that I'm a true Scot — just like Aussies, we have a love of alcohol that is etched into our national identity in indelible ink. Maybe it's the depressing weather, a history of oppression, or our reputation for sporting catastrophe that has driven us to drink. Or perhaps it's just that we're a nation built on booze. We've produced some of the most significant inventions in modern history: the steam engine, penicillin (the Aussies may have had the smarts to bring it to market, but it was Sir Alexander Fleming, a Scot, who discovered it), the telephone, and the television. But the export for which we're most renowned, and which fuels the national economy, is whisky.

Despite Mum's impressive malt collection, I've never enjoyed the 'water of life'. I can't stomach the taste — even of the really good stuff. Over the years, I've made up for this aberration by embracing practically every other form of alcohol known to man. So it's with some trepidation that I head home booze-free to a country that has turned binge drinking into an art form.

In the airport departure lounge, I have to stop myself from ordering a beer at the bar. This time last year, Kath and I were drinking champagne at this very spot, toasting the start of a five-week trip to Spain and Italy via Edinburgh. It strikes me that drinking has historically been the way I mark the start of all my holidays; it's the signal that work is officially over and relaxation time has begun.

I order a lemonade instead. It doesn't feel the same.

Last year, during my ten days in Edinburgh, I don't think I went one day without having a drink. As in Australia, in Scotland bonding tends to be accompanied by alcohol — and when you live on the other side of the world, a boozy homecoming is practically a legal requirement. Every catch-up with friends, family, and former colleagues is toasted with alcohol.

I was particularly nervous about telling Fiona that this visit would be a sober one. Last time I came home, we went out to a nightclub we used to frequent in our university days, drinking tequila shots and dancing to The Smiths till 3.00 a.m. She assures me that my sobriety is not a concern, and that we'll have fun together regardless of what we're drinking, pointing out that she's had two children and has more experience of abstaining from alcohol for long periods of time than I do.

I'm still apprehensive. This time, those reunions won't be toasted with glasses of wine; it'll be cups of tea and glasses of juice. But my friend Ruth tells me that she's quite relieved that I won't be drinking this time around. 'I have to steel myself for your visits. I always associate you coming home with a massive piss-up,' she says. 'The worst hangover I've ever had was after one of your homecomings and we stayed out till 2.00 a.m. I had to work the next morning and I was very sick.'

Maybe it's not being Scottish that makes my trips home drunken affairs. Maybe it's just me.

However, some Edinburgh friends see it differently. The boys from my old paper *The Daily Record* vow to steer me off course, telling me that it's bordering on treacherous not to drink. It seems I'll dilute some of my Scottishness if I'm drinking orange juice. People never tire of telling me I've already lost my accent — which, after ten years in Melbourne, I've come to think of as 'Scotralian' — so refusing a drink will be further evidence of my defection. Somehow I'll be letting my country down if I don't get steamin', pished, swallied, blootered, bladdered, reekin', hammered, wellied, leathered, fleein', fu', steamboats, guttered, wrecked, mortal, buckled, mingin', bleezin', muntered, fullyit, arseholed, or oot o' it. The Eskimos might have 50 words for snow, but we've got at least 450 for being drunk.

I spend the long flight thinking about home. When I arrive, Mum and I will traditionally crack open a bottle of wine and stay up as long as my jetlag allows, catching up on lost time. This trip will be different, and I'm quite looking forward to it. Time with family is so precious; I'm going to enjoy not having it clouded by the haze of tipsiness.

I grew up surrounded by alcohol. My parents loved a drink, as did most of my friends' parents. Family get-togethers were usually fairly boozy affairs. I loved it when the oldies got a bit squiffy — what child doesn't like seeing their parents laugh, dance, and be silly?

As older teenagers, Neil and I were allowed to drink at home. Mum and Dad felt that if we were going to drink, at least they could maintain some supervision if we did it under their roof, rather than sneaking out behind their backs and putting ourselves in risky situations. (What they didn't know was that we were doing both.) Our house became the mustering point for our friends before we'd all hit the town. It was also the crash pad; some Sunday mornings there were so many doonas in our lounge room that it was hard to tell how many bodies lay beneath. My friends loved my parents' parties so much that even when I moved to the other side of the world, they'd still turn up for their annual Boxing Day bash, cram into my old bedroom, and call me in varying states of intoxication to tell me what I was missing out on.

But now, as I prepare to return home sober, with Jon Currie's words still fresh in my mind, I start to think of these events in a different light. Was this the start of my 'pre-malignant addiction'? Did I cultivate it from an early age, learning through my parents' liberal attitude to drinking that alcohol is what makes life fun?

When I caught up with John Rogerson, chief executive of the Australian Drug Foundation, shortly after he read the story about my binge drinking, he was keen to know if my parents drank when I was growing up. I told him they weren't massive drinkers, but they liked to have a good time — and that our house did latterly become a bit of a party house. He told me research is increasingly showing that children mimic their parents' drinking habits, and that this can influence the relationship they have with alcohol in later life. I can't help being a bit cynical about this. My parents may have influenced me, but it's not the only reason I drink. And I know just as many people who grew up in families where booze was strictly off-limits, rebelled at the first possible opportunity, and went on to drink heavily. Drinking habits, as I'm learning, cannot easily be attributed to any one factor. But what I now know for sure is that when there's a genetic predisposal to dependency, binge drinking is a risky pastime.

My granddad had a drinking problem. His should have been a cautionary tale, but I've been able to dismiss any link between my drinking and his because we're not blood relatives. He was the only father Mum ever knew, but he was Gran's second husband, marrying her when Mum was ten. I know that his drinking has hurt our family. The details are sketchy — I think my parents tried to shield Neil and me from much of it. Now, as I return home sober, with a clear head and more insight into the nature of addiction than I've ever had, I'm ready to know more.

Granddad was a handsome, gentle man, who wore a kilt more often than he wore trousers. A true Highlander, he was born in the depths of an unforgiving Isle of Skye winter, in the village of Uig. He had a full head of white hair and a bushy moustache — and an enormous capacity for love. He never tired of telling me and Neil (his namesake) how much we meant to him. But his declarations usually happened when he was drunk. And he was drunk a lot. Sometimes his phone calls were incoherent. It was like listening to a sailor trying to shush a baby: there was lots of gruff oohing and aahing and whispered pet names, but not a whole lot of sense.

As a teenager, I found these calls mortifying. I hated explaining my granddad's 'situation' to my friends. When he'd talk to me in a baby voice, calling me 'Jilly' or 'wee scone', and promising to come and see me soon, my face would flush. I'd rush to get off the phone and put Mum on. It's funny how your priorities change when you're no longer shackled by the pursuit of acceptance and the aching need to be normal; I'd give anything to have one more conversation with him. He could call me whatever he liked.

Granddad was never an aggressive or violent drunk. He was rarely maudlin. For the most part, he was sentimental and sweet. But even the most good-natured addict will eventually hurt the ones they love. One night, after a long session at his local, the barman told Granddad that he'd had one too many, confiscating his car keys. A fellow drinker, observing this exchange, later offered to drive him home and make sure he got back to his wife safely. The man took him home, but stole the car. Another time, Granddad told Gran that he was nipping out to buy a paper. She didn't see him for three days. When he returned, paper in hand, he explained, 'There was a long queue.' It's a story that took on folklore status in our family — an amusing anecdote that turned a disease into a quaint character foible. It's this type of story about Granddad that I remember vividly. Perhaps the passing of time has blurred the bleaker parts of those years, leaving only the harmless stories in sharp focus. I know that the reality was uglier.

A few nights after I arrive home, Mum and I are curled up in armchairs in her living room, our traditional glasses of wine replaced with cups of tea. I ask if she'll tell me the story of Granddad's drinking. She speaks softly as she tells me how her parents disintegrated.

It was the late 1980s, and Granddad had been drinking a lot. He'd been disappearing, often for days at a time. A dam can only take so much pressure before it bursts. One afternoon, Mum walked into her parents' flat on the south side of Edinburgh to find her mother sitting alone in the kitchen, in her favourite chair beside the fire, her face drained of colour. 'I knew straight away that something was really wrong. She stood up, burst into tears, and just collapsed in my arms: "I can't do it anymore; I just can't do it." She was sobbing and shaking.'

Mum had never seen this proud Highland-born woman so distressed. Gran was inconsolable. She needed the sort of help Mum couldn't give her. They went to the family doctor, who made an emergency appointment at the Royal Edinburgh — a psychiatric hospital. When they got there, Gran made a plea to the admitting doctor. 'Mum was begging, *begging* this man, "Please take me in, take me in. I need to be here." She was exhausted. She couldn't cope.

She just needed peace. When I left her there, in a locked psychiatric ward full of geriatrics, that was the worst day of my life.'

Mum's voice breaks a little. She pauses, staring straight ahead. She takes a deep breath that seems to cause her physical pain. 'The second-worst day of my life was telling Dad that Mum wasn't coming home, that she couldn't live with him anymore. That was the only time in my entire life when he raised his voice to me. He just couldn't comprehend how his drinking was hurting her. But the stress of not knowing where he was or when he was coming home, of not being able to rely on anything he said — it was too much. And she was tired of lying and hiding this from people. She was tired of making excuses to his work and to family about him.'

Granddad's boss, at the electrical-engineering firm where he worked, knew that Grandad had a drinking problem but didn't want to sack him, fearful of the maelstrom it might trigger. Instead, he sent him to a doctor, who ran some tests. The doctor couldn't believe he was still alive. Still, Granddad kept drinking. Mum persuaded him to go to an Alcoholics Anonymous meeting. 'We were sitting around in a circle and everyone was introducing themselves — "I'm Pamela, I'm an alcoholic," and so on. And the man said, "We've got a new member tonight. Neil, would you like to say anything?" I was holding his hand, and he just shook his head. I knew then that we'd lost. He physically couldn't bring himself to say that he had a problem.'

Gran was in hospital for six months. 'For a long time, she didn't smile. She was just blank-faced when I'd go in to see her; she'd be sitting in a chair, staring into space. One day, I went in and there was a gardener outside, and he'd lit a bonfire. Mum was staring at the smoke rising up, and she said, "That's where they burn the bodies. That's where I'm going. To the crematorium." That broke my heart. She thought that would be the best answer, to just not be alive anymore.'

Gran's nervous breakdown was compounded by guilt. She worried about being a burden, and about the effect that her illness was having on her family. The weight of it all only exacerbated her depression. She'd been divorced once already, at a time when women in unhappy marriages were expected to grin and bear it. The shame of another failed marriage would be devastating. But at the root of all her sadness was the fact that she missed her husband dreadfully. Logically, she knew that he was the reason she'd fallen off a cliff, but in her heart he was the rope that could pull her back up again. 'The great tragedy of it all was they loved each other. They couldn't live with each other and they couldn't live without each other,' Mum says.

Slowly, Gran started to improve. 'One day I walked in and Mum was smiling. I burst into tears because I knew I had my mum back. She looked at me and said, "I know it's corny, but today is the first day of the rest of my life." Of course, there was worse to come, but we believed it at the time.' The doctors wouldn't discharge Gran from hospital into the care of the man they believed was aggravating her condition, so she came to stay with us for a while. Then she moved to be with Mum's older sister Kitty, in Stockport, just outside of Manchester. Granddad moved to Inverness, and they sold their Edinburgh flat. But Gran pined for her husband. It wasn't long before she went back to him, heading north to Inverness, to what Mum describes as a 'poky wee flat'. 'He'd be out drinking and she'd just sit in front of the fire. She was miserable. He was a good man. He loved her so much; he loved her to bits. He'd stop drinking and I'd pray, I would literally pray, that this would be it. That he'd stop. But he always went back.'

Gran's health gradually began to deteriorate again. Eventually, she required constant care and was moved to a nursing home. She died on 6 January 1992. 'Granddad really just carried on as before. He did try to moderate his drinking, but he missed her so much that he found it almost impossible. I visited him a few times, and he was always so happy to see me, but I knew that nothing I did would change him because he really did not want to stop drinking. He did not acknowledge that he had a problem, and eventually he died.' That was on 20 August 1999.

Mum's worn out by the time she's finished. We're both in tears. The decisions she had to make to help look after the people who raised her are unimaginable. That she was able to function while coping with that trauma, let alone maintain a marriage and care for two children, ensuring that they had a normal life, fills me with a love for her that no words can explain fully. And at the heart of that tragedy: alcohol. A drug I have enjoyed with cavalier abandon simply because it's legal.

I GO FOR a night out with Fiona and Lisa, my oldest and dearest friends. We've been pals since primary school. This time, without alcohol, it's different. It's better. It's wonderful to catch up on their news.

After dinner, we weigh up where to go next. A pub? A nightclub? But all we really want to do is talk. I drive us back to Fiona's house and, while they drink wine, I sip peppermint tea. We chat until well past 2.00 a.m. These are the memories that will keep me warm in my old age.

We talk about drinking, too. That's been happening a lot lately. My sobriety, already old-hat in Melbourne, sparks new conversations here — not the usual, 'You were so pished last night!' war stories, but a real conversation, about how much we drink, why we drink, and how Scotland is a nation with a drinking problem. Granddad's story is not uncommon: nearly everyone knows someone who has struggled with alcoholism, whether it's a neighbour, a relative, a colleague, or a friend. I'm amazed at how common these tales are, and wonder if it's always been this way and we've just never talked about it, or if I've been too busy getting drunk to notice.

The next morning I hear Scotland's first minister, Alex Salmond, interviewed on radio about Gerry Rafferty, the singer-songwriter who wrote 'Baker Street' and 'Stuck in the Middle with You'. Rafferty died in January from liver failure, after decades of heavy drinking. Salmond talks about Rafferty's 'enormous talent', and adds, 'Unfortunately, like many people in Scotland, he fell victim to the bottle.' It's a throwaway line, but it says so much. Scots poetise alcohol, turning it into a predator poised to devour the unwitting; the 'demon drink' can be our mortal enemy, but also our closest friend. Our national bard, Robert Burns, thought to have died from complications related to excessive drinking, wrote the epic 'Tam o' Shanter', a gothic tale of a man who spends too long at a public house and is plagued by nightmarish visions on his way home. But it's his many poems celebrating alcohol, including one that posits 'freedom an' whisky gang thegither', that we cling to most as proof that our tradition and cultural identity are inextricably linked to booze.

On a radio phone-in the day after the interview with Alex Salmond, the topic is the nation's record of sporting failure. The presenter asks what Olympic sport Scotland would win gold in; the resounding response from callers is, of course, drinking. The host laughs and makes a quip about our legendary boozing reputation. But Scotland's unenviable title of the sick man of Europe is no joke. In the country responsible for the deep-fried Mars Bar, obesity and heart-disease rates are soaring. Smoking is not yet out of fashion, with 27 per cent of men hooked, compared to 21 per cent in the rest of the United Kingdom, and 18 per cent in Australia. Life expectancy in Scotland is two years fewer than in Great Britain's other home nations. But the most insidious killer of all is booze: 15 of the 20 areas in the United Kingdom with the highest number of alcohol-related deaths are in Scotland. In some parts of Glasgow, men are lucky if they live beyond their fifties. Over the last two decades, liver-cirrhosis rates have increased by 450 per cent, at a time when rates in most of Western Europe have been falling. A recent analysis of alcohol sales found that the average Scottish adult is knocking back the equivalent of 46 bottles of vodka every year. If health experts in Australia are worried about the binge-drinking culture Down Under, they should take a trip to Scotland to see how much worse things could be. The population is four times smaller than Australia's, but every year the same number of people — more than 3000 — die from booze-related causes. As a race, we are drinking ourselves to death.

Public concern is so heightened that the once-sacred tradition of happy hour has been banned in Scottish pubs. Buy-one-get-one-free deals in off-licences have also been outlawed. And in a sign that the party truly is over, Scotland looks set to become the first country in Europe to introduce a minimum price for alcohol. A bill to be put before the Scottish Parliament in 2012 aims to end systemic discounting, which has allowed retailers to sell a bottle of cider more cheaply than a bottle of water. It will mean that a unit of alcohol cannot be sold below a set price (thought to be around 45 pence) and will make stronger drinks, associated with heavy drinking, less affordable. Announcing the legislation, health secretary Nicola Sturgeon vowed, 'It is time for Scotland to win its battle with the booze.'*

I arrange to meet a woman on the front lines of this battle. Evelyn Gillan is the head of Alcohol Focus Scotland, a charity set up to reduce alcohol harm and create a culture where moderate drinking is the norm. It's a daunting task in a country with whisky as one of its most lucrative exports, contributing £3 billion a year to the national

---

* The Scottish Parliament passed the Alcohol (Minimum Pricing) Bill in May 2012, setting the minimum price for a unit of alcohol at 50 pence, meaning that the cheapest bottle of wine would be £4.69 and a four-pack of lager would cost at least £3.52. The Scotch Whisky Association and the European Spirits Organisation fought the legislation, claiming it breached EU trade rules, in a lengthy legal battle that dragged on until 2017 when the UK's Supreme Court rejected the case, saying minimum pricing was, 'proportionate means of achieving a legitimate aim'. The minimum pricing Act came into effect in May 2018. Alcohol sales in Scotland fell by 8 per cent after the law was introduced.

economy. But when we catch up for coffee in Edinburgh's New Town, I realise that if you're going to fight a war, you'd want Evelyn Gillan in your corner. She speaks quickly, in urgent tones, with a broad Scots accent. Immaculately dressed and with her hair in a neat bob, she doesn't look much like a warrior — but make no mistake, she's locked in combat. Her enemy: the alcohol industry. When she describes the industry as 'disease vectors', I laugh. She doesn't. 'Seriously, it's a hazardous, harmful product. It's a drug, and we've allowed the producers of that hazardous product unfettered access to young people. Now we're concerned when we see 12-year-olds being hospitalised on a Friday night. Why should we be surprised, when we actually look at what we've allowed to happen over the last 30 years?'

Just as Robin Room argues that a reputation for binge drinking is part of Australia's national myth, fuelled partly by market forces, Gillan says Scotland's drinking problem is a corporate-born epidemic. Alcohol consumption in the 1960s was relatively low, around five litres of alcohol per person over the age of 15 per year. Today, it's more than 12 litres. 'Increasingly, we have to name and identify the role of the big multinationals in fuelling this epidemic, instead of just saying, "It's our culture — we all love our drink." That's not happened by accident. There's very specific action that's been taken with deregulation, liberalisation, proliferation of new alcohol products, and massive spends on advertising.' Gillan says that booze has, since the 1970s, become cheaper, more heavily marketed, and more readily available. 'When I was young, you couldn't afford to drink at home. A litre bottle of vodka was the equivalent of £35. If you had anything in the house, it was for New Year's Eve. At the supermarket, alcohol and tobacco used to be screened off behind a separate section. There's been a big push by the industry to make alcohol an ordinary commodity, and available 24 hours a day, seven days a week.'

There's a quiet fury beneath her words. She talks about the need to 'protect' young people from the 'normalisation' of drinking, led by an industry bombarding them with alcohol advertising at sporting events, at music festivals, and, increasingly, through social media, where there are no restrictions on how to market alcohol products. She says that not only is this type of viral marketing big bang for the industry buck, but also that Facebook or Bebo groups which promote funky new drinks create a sense of belonging in an audience desperate for peer acceptance. Young people are much more likely to pay attention to brand messages if the recommendation comes directly from their friends.

Internal marketing documents from British beer giant Carling, obtained during a 2009 House of Commons Health Select Committee inquiry into alcohol advertising, revealed that the purpose of the company's sponsorship of music festivals was to 'build the image of the brand and recruit young male drinkers'. The document stated: 'More people are attending live music than ever before. FACT. Which is great for Carling as beer and live music go hand in hand. FACT.' The company sought to make Carling 'the first choice for festival virgins', and enhanced its brand during the event through a range of promotions, including handing out free tents, and offering a campsite morning-delivery service of a can of Carling and a newspaper. 'Great way to start the day!' the documents stated.

This form of insidious marketing, Gillan says, is a powerful way to attract new drinkers. 'What we're trying to do is turn that around and start protecting people from alcohol marketing, and empowering young people — like the tobacco-truth campaigns, where once young people have got access to information about how the industry is trying to manipulate them and dupe them, they say, "I don't think so."' Gillan says that she wasn't always this combative. But as the industry fights moves towards regulation —

particularly minimum price, which alcohol companies claim won't reduce problem drinking and will penalise the majority of Scots, who drink responsibly — she's been forced to defend herself. 'I've had personal attacks. I've been called a neo-prohibitionist. I think my current nickname within the industry is Dr Evil Glam. I've been shouted at in rooms. If they can't win the argument, they attack the organisation. The industry is fantastically organised; very successful lobbyists. It's a David-and-Goliath battle.'

As an example, she cites the Scotch Whisky Association, one of the most vocal opponents of minimum price legislation, which has appealed to national sentiment by claiming that Scotland's most iconic export will be threatened by the move. But the group is not what it seems. Far from being a collective of local distilleries fighting for Scottish jobs, its 56 members include some of the world's largest multinational alcohol companies. It was until recently chaired by Diageo, a global spirits giant that produces brands such as Smirnoff, Johnnie Walker, and Baileys. Gillan claims that the industry is fundamentally opposed to any moves to reduce consumption because if people drink less, these companies make less money.

The influence of the multinationals' massive marketing spend, says Gillan, is contributing to a shift in the way young people are drinking in parts of Europe that have, until recently, not seen the alcohol-related social consequences felt so keenly in the United Kingdom and Australia. In France, Spain, and Italy, where historically alcohol was drunk in the Mediterranean tradition, mainly with food, more young people are now drinking recreationally. 'They're drinking branded beers and spirits that were never associated with their cultures. Again, the industry's got massive presences in these countries. What the public-health people are saying is that if you go to Madrid or other main cities, that's where you start to see major public drunkenness for the first time. It will be sad if it goes that way because the way they traditionally drink just shows you that it's possible to create a culture where people don't think it's cool to be plastered.'

I'm reminded of an evening with Kath, during our jaunt around Europe last year. We were in a bar in Venice, watching Germany and Spain in the World Cup semi-final. After the game, hundreds of young people spilled out of bars and restaurants, and we found ourselves sitting at the foot of some steps in a piazza, drinking bottled beer and people-watching. Some were drinking; many were not. What struck me was how convivial the atmosphere was. The throng grew, and there was a bit of jostling as people pushed to get through the crowd. But there was no trouble. I've spent a lot of time in the city centres of Melbourne and Edinburgh on Friday and Saturday nights, and there's always that underlying threat of menace. It's a tinderbox just waiting for a match. But in Venice, I felt completely safe. The difference, I think, is that their drinking seemed to be incidental. Ours is often the whole point of the evening.

Before I leave, I ask Gillan where she'd like to see Scotland in ten years. On her wish list is greater regulation so that alcohol costs more and is less accessible, and children are not 'saturated' with drinking messages. 'If we had all of that, then I wouldn't expect the number of people to die. I would expect half our jails to be empty because 50 per cent of our prisoners were drunk at the time of the offence. Our accident and emergency departments would not be warzones at the weekend. I'd like low alcohol consumption to be the norm, and I'd like those who choose not to drink to be supported in their choice.'

After we say our goodbyes, I reflect on her crusade. It's an admirable one. But I'm not sure I share her view that the alcohol industry carries so much of the blame for youth binge drinking. Teenagers are risk-takers; getting drunk is about testing boundaries and experimenting. I started drinking at 13 and, unless the industry marketing machine was so sophisticated that I didn't realise I was being targeted, I don't think advertising played much, if any, role in why I did it. Although today's teenager might be bombarded with colourful alcopops designed to appeal to an unsophisticated palate, when I was young there weren't any sweet-tasting drinks to mask the foul taste of hard liquor. It didn't deter me.

I walk back to Mum's flat via Bruntsfield Links, a green space popular with tourists for being one of the earliest known locations where the game of golf was played, sometime around the 15th century. For me it brings back teenage memories of lazy afternoons lying in the sunshine with friends, drinking a carryout and smoking fags. I throw my bag on the ground and lie down, resting my head on it. Not much has changed. To my left a group of teenagers, boys and girls aged 18 or 19, are sprawled out in a circle, drinking cider and playing guitars. I can smell hash. They're approached by a German man riding a unicycle, and they collapse into giggles. Before long, everyone is giving the unicycle a go.

Behind me, another group of girls, who look about 15 or 16, are talking about T in the Park, Scotland's biggest music festival. The T stands for Tennent's, a Scottish brewery and the festival's major sponsor since it began in 1994, my last year of high school. Last time I went it was 1995, and The Prodigy, Supergrass, and The Verve were among the headline acts. I was pissed for two days, but I didn't drink Tennent's. The girls are excited because they've discovered vodka pouches, single-serve soft packs of spirits that they plan to smuggle past security in their wellies. The conversation shifts to the weekend just gone. 'I was absolutely steamin'. I was, like, still drunk the next day at two o'clock. Then I went out the next night, got home at 5.30, and Sarah's parents woke us up at, like, nine o'clock. Then I totally had this rash cos I was just, like, so rundown. For two nights I'd had, like, six hours asleep, and I just spewed.' All three girls burst out laughing.

When I get back to the flat, I start to sift through my childhood. Mum's living room is strewn with bags and boxes of stuff I've collected over the years, retrieved from the attic of our family home last year after my parents sold up. This is the first chance I've had to go through it. There are letters from pen pals in Denmark and Australia, and certificates for swimming, skiing, and tap dancing, and a Brownie tea-making badge. I find the order of service for Granddad's funeral, and a small piece of card that says 'cord number 3' — a pallbearer's instructions. There are several editions of 'Paw's Fitba Talk', a monthly newsletter Dad wrote for me about Scottish football when I was living in New Zealand: twelve editions of pure love. I laugh at handwritten notes Fiona passed to me during history class, her acerbic assessment of our teachers even funnier today given she's now a teacher herself. There are literally hundreds of photographs of the two of us. We're pissed in many of them.

When Fiona comes over for dinner and to look through the boxes, I bring up the more outrageous moments of our teenage years — the time we sneaked vodka from my parents' drinks cabinet at lunchtime and giggled our way through choir practice, or the day my folks came back unexpectedly early from a golf day in St Andrews, and we had to hide beer cans down the back of the couch and tip ashtrays into our pockets. She claims amnesia, joking the next day on Facebook that she's seeking the services of a libel lawyer. But my diaries don't lie. It seems that I was drunk for pretty much the whole of the '90s and most of the 2000s.

One diary entry stands out more than most: October 1992. I was 16.

I feel like I'm growing up too fast. I go out every weekend to pubs and get totally drunk. I have to stop drinking because according to everyone (all guys incidentally) I'm a much nicer person when I'm sober. But it's a vicious circle. If I'm drunk I talk to people and meet people with confidence in myself and they tend not to like me but if I stay sober I don't talk to people or meet people because I'm too shy and they won't be able to find out if I'm nice or not. I just want to die. My life is so shit just now. I hate school and I don't even have anything to look forward to at the weekend anymore.

I stare at the words, the handwriting so messy and childlike. The melodrama makes me smile. It was, and sometimes still is, my forte. But the underlying point is hard to ignore: for 20 years I've been drinking like this. And I was questioning it even at the start. I drank for confidence and to chat to guys. It left me feeling depressed, dissatisfied, and bored. How much has changed? I think about Jon Currie's offer to test my brain and decide I'm going to do it. Maybe it will help me to understand how much of my adult personality — my anxiety and bouts of depression, my impulsivity and short temper — have been caused by getting drunk as a teenager. The results might not be pleasant, but I need to know.

July

MUM AND I are taking a road trip. I've travelled to every state and territory in Australia, an island continent that could fit Scotland 97 times, but to my shame I've seen very little of my compact homeland. Despite spending the first 25 years of my life in Edinburgh, I rarely ventured past Glasgow, which is less than an hour's drive away. Yet the yearning to see more of my country grows stronger with every year I'm away. My mum's family were Highlanders and, although she grew up in Edinburgh, she spent many happy summers with her aunt in a small village called Whitebridge, on the south shore of Loch Ness. She wants to take me there; I can't wait. Perhaps by touring these historic areas I'll get some clues as to why drinking is such an integral part of my national identity.

The morning we set out is the kind of Scottish summer's day that has to be seen to be believed. It's ten degrees and *dreich* — a Scottish term, invented because no other word could adequately capture the unique brand of soggy, grey misery known only to our shores. It's pronounced with emphasis on the guttural sound of the last two letters, and Mum maintains that it should be spat out like an unwelcome taste, as if in direct reference to the weather it represents. As we drive out of Edinburgh, towards Fife, on the city bypass, rain teems down in sheets. One of Scotland's most iconic landmarks, the Forth Rail Bridge is all but obscured, its majestic peaks shrouded under low-lying cloud. The sky ahead is gunmetal grey as we drive north into Perthshire. Douglas firs line the road, their proud silhouettes stretching in neat rows all the way up the ranges to the west. I can smell the pine wafting through the air vents, and immediately I'm back in my parents' living room on Christmas Eve, sitting cross-legged in the dark before a tree straining under the weight of tinsel and toilet paper–tube Santas. If ever I feel alone, all I have to do is remember that smell.

At times, the rain falls so hard that I can barely see the car in front of me. I'm annoyed that this precious time with Mum should be so rudely blighted. But this is home; it's always been this way. Ask a Scotsman what he calls six weeks of rain, and he'll reply, 'Summer.' Scotland is often at her most dramatic when enveloped in mist or drizzle. Ours is a history of struggle, a past steeped in bloody battles and violent uprisings. It's only fitting that the weather should match that.

We arrive in Pitlochry, gateway to the Highlands, and head up a narrow road to the hotel where we'll be spending the night. When I see it, I think Mum must be having a laugh. As if travelling through the Highlands — where there are more pubs and distilleries than people — completely sober isn't enough of a challenge, Mum has booked us into a brewery for the night. The hotel, which has been a travellers' rest since 1695, boasts some of the region's finest ales, with evocative names such as Braveheart and Old Remedial, none of which I'll be enjoying. Over lunch, Mum giggles, telling me, 'I wanted it to be authentic for you,' as she clinks her delicious-looking amber ale against my sad glass of Diet Coke. When I ask her why we Scots don't always look each other in the eye when we say *slàinte mhath* (the equivalent of 'cheers', meaning 'your very good health'), as is customary in Australia, she's not sure, but suggests perhaps it's because the priority is to keep an eye on your drink so you don't spill any.

In keeping with the tone, we decide to while away the wet afternoon in a distillery. We trundle down a snaky single-track road until we arrive at Edradour, the smallest distillery in Scotland. This is the very type of business the alcohol industry claims will face closure should a minimum price for alcohol be introduced. That would be a sad day indeed. This place is charming beyond words. Unlike the larger operations, which use computerised systems to mass-produce a drink that has a global market, Edradour is the last distillery in Scotland where you can see malt whisky made by hand. They use the same traditional copper-pot stills as the bigger distilleries, but they're much smaller, the largest one holding just 800 gallons of whisky — which, to my mind, still seems like an enormous amount of Scotch. But here at Edradour, our kilted tour guide tells us, they produce in a year what the big distilleries make in a week: just 15 casks. The whisky sits in the warehouse in its cask for ten years. About a quarter of each barrel will evaporate over that time. This is called 'the angels' share'. It's not hard to see how we developed a national obsession with drinking; the language of alcohol in Scotland is heavenly. We pay the amber drop so much reverence; is it any wonder I've grown up to be such a prolific drinker?

Our guide tells us that, unlike wine, malt whisky doesn't mature in the bottle, so 'if you buy it, drink it'. When the tray of sample drams is handed around, I don't have to be told what to do. I accept the glass, nose it — breathing in the fumes of a drink that, despite Mum's marketing campaign, has always smelled to me like drain cleaner — and pour it, discreetly, into her glass. Even with my unpatriotic palate, I still feel like I'm missing out. Any other time I would down that dram, just because it's there; refusing a free drink just isn't in me. And at 63 per cent alcohol, if nothing else it would warm me up.

When we wake the following day, it's still overcast, but the rain has stopped. I stick my head out the window of our top-floor room (a place that isn't without charm but, with its wall-to-wall tartan, invokes a claustrophobic sense of being trapped inside a shortbread tin) and inhale the cleansing air. I feel energised in one breath. We head out early and sit on the banks of the River Tummel, a mesmerising, fast-flowing expanse of water. The salmon making their way to spawning grounds upstream are battling a strong current, occasionally leaping out of the water on their epic journey. I watch in admiration, knowing how hard it is to swim against a tide that tries so intently to pull you back the way you came.

To get a bird's-eye perspective of the area, we head up to Queen's View. This scenic lookout was made famous by a visit from Queen Victoria in 1866, but is actually thought to have been named after Queen Isabella, wife of Robert the Bruce. It's a sight fit for a queen: lush greenery hugs the banks of a loch as clear and still as glass, stretching all the way into the Glencoe mountains to the west. It's staggeringly beautiful. Other than the electricity pylons and the narrow road that winds through the hills, there's little sign that the landscape has changed in centuries. It's hard to believe a place so tranquil has such a savage history.

At dinner, I'm faced with a dilemma. The traditional Scottish menu offers few options that haven't been fried, baked, stewed, poached, or otherwise doused in alcohol. There's venison with a port-and-cranberry jus, salmon in a chardonnay-and-chive cream sauce, duck with black cherries and blackcurrant liqueur, and an Angus fillet of beef in a whisky sauce. It feels almost traitorous to go for boring old chicken, or vegetarian lasagne, so I pick the local salmon, hoping that the cooking process will render the alcohol content of my meal negligible. As we tuck in, I feel conspicuous not drinking with my meal. Like us, most of the people in this quaint dining room, with its tartan tablecloths and pictures of native birds and fish, are visitors to the area. They're marking their holidays by drinking bottles of wine and sampling the local beer and malt whisky. I feel as if I'm not getting the full Highland experience by sipping water.

Mum says it's funny that I feel so exposed when it wasn't that long ago the sight of a woman drinking would have scandalised the locals. In the 1960s, when she was young, Scottish women didn't drink in public. Drinking out of a bottle would be enough to classify you as a loose woman. Pub windows would often be blacked out, or have the lower halves frosted, to prevent people from looking in. This, Mum says, was partly to protect children from witnessing the effects of the 'demon drink', but also so that men could enjoy a beer without their nosy womenfolk knowing where they were. 'It was a man's right to drink and not be seen,' Mum says.

It sounds archaic. But then I compare it to what my friend Joanne told me recently about the way some Scottish women carry on in pubs these days. Having worked as a manager in the Glasgow pub trade for more than ten years, she's seen it all. On Old Firm match days — a football derby between archenemies Rangers and Celtic that has a shocking history of sectarian violence — she's seen alcohol-fuelled fights become full-scale riots. Predominantly, they involve men. But what really shocks her is the way that some women are now behaving. You would think that the reunion of a '90s boy band would be a sedate affair, but when English pop group Take That staged a comeback tour in June, the streets of Glasgow were overrun with wasted middle-aged women. Many had been on marathon drinking sessions before the gig even started; some were so boozed, they collapsed. Others flashed their boobs at passing cars and urinated in the street. Joanne says that they were feral in the pub after the show: verbally abusing bar staff and generally being obnoxious. It's hard to say what's more offensive — women being branded as sluts for daring to have a drink in a man's domain, or women getting so tanked that they relieve themselves in the gutter and pick fights with strangers.

After dinner, instead of setting up camp in the bar, Mum and I climb the twisty stairs to our bedroom and drink cups of tea while we huddle together over my laptop, watching *Downton Abbey* on DVD. It's not very rock 'n' roll, but these moments shared with Mum are special.

Throughout our journey, the scenery continues to amaze us. We pass Ardverikie House, more famously known as Glenbogle Castle in the BBC series *Monarch of the Glen*. Its fairytale turrets are even more impressive in real life. We travel miles without seeing another car, stopping occasionally to admire the stately homes and grand buildings nestled among the forests. In Australia, 1950s bungalows and austere office blocks are often heritage-listed attractions; in Scotland, centuries-old properties are so plentiful that many don't even merit a mention on the map.

As we get closer to Whitebridge, we mistakenly take a trip down a gravelly road that leads us deep into another Highland estate. Our only companions are sheep, ambling across the unsealed road. We pass another grand residence, perched next to a river that runs under a stone bridge and into an expansive inlet flanked by mountains. It's the kind of scenery that's hard to comprehend: a view so impressive that it feels like a guilty pleasure just being there. I get out of the car and absorb the serene silence, not a soul in sight. The stress of city life, the redundancies, my troubling thoughts about addiction, and my past and my future, all drift away from me like mist. After months of noise, finally some peace.

WE ARRIVE TO spend the night in a lovely bed and breakfast, where the owner recommends we try the pub at the end of the road. Mum tells him that I don't drink. 'I don't drink just now,' I clarify, perhaps a smidgen too hastily. After all this time, it's weird that I still don't want to be judged by strangers as a boring teetotaller. Living so far from my homeland, I feel my Scottishness is being slowly chipped away with each year that passes. I worry that my abstinence only highlights my foreignness.

We wake to see a family of pheasants pecking around outside our bedroom window. The stillness of the Highlands is soothing. I feel my body and mind relaxing into the endless space around us. We head off to visit Aunty Cissie's house, an old croft at the end of a single-track road, nestled in a thick forest. The trees were knee-high saplings when Mum was a girl. She remembers running in and out of them with her brother and sister during their school holidays. Cissie, who Mum always called Atta because as a child she couldn't pronounce 'aunty', died in 1964. Mum has been back to visit her home a couple of times, but not for many years. As we stand outside the house, an elderly neighbour, with ruddy cheeks and billowing cotton-wool hair, approaches. He greets us with a broad smile. When Mum tells him who she is, he bundles her into an embrace and says he knew of Aunt Atta. His nephew now owns the house Mum spent so much of her childhood in. He asks if we want a dram. 'I find it very lubricating,' he says. 'It eases the joints. Very good medicine.' We politely decline. It's ten o'clock in the morning.

Everywhere we go, we're greeted by strangers as if we're family. My Scottish accent, tinged with that upward Aussie inflection, returns with full force. It's no longer 'yes' but 'aye', 'cannae' not 'can't', 'tatties' rather than 'potatoes'. The scenery grows more breathtaking with every bend rounded. Driving near Whitebridge, we see deer grazing on a hillside, just metres from us. As we pull over, they stop eating and look up, the stag staring directly at me, transfixed. Later, at the Falls of Foyers, a waterfall that feeds into Loch Ness, something unexpected happens: the sights, smells, and sounds of my homeland prove too much. As the water thunders, I look across the canopy of trees to a deep gorge, which rises up to a cliff top lined with pine trees. It's a view of such uncompromising beauty that I find myself in tears. As I take in the vivid green fields and the storybook mountains beyond, the emotion pours out of me. I am home, at peace, and totally alive. I have a sense of my place in the world that seems to ground my soul to the Highland soil. Mum puts an arm around my shoulder and I rest my head against hers. We look on in awe at the show our country is putting on for us. I'm so lucky.

Later, as the late-evening sun sets and the horizon turns to fairy floss, we crank up the volume on Frankie Miller's version of Dougie MacLean's 'Caledonia', an unofficial Scottish national anthem, and belt it out as we drive through twisty roads carved into a glen that stretches on for miles. '*Let me tell you that I love you / That I think about you all the time / Caledonia, you're calling me / And now I'm going home.*' In that moment, fingers intertwined, we are the only two people on the planet. I worried that a homecoming without alcohol would make my national identity disappear, but I've never felt more Scottish. I know now that national pride is not built on alcohol. I worried that not drinking would prevent me from reconnecting with the ones I love, but my heart's so full there's no room for booze.

WHEN WE RETURN from the Highlands, it's not long before we're back on the road. This time, we're off to the Lake District for Mum's sister Kitty's 70th birthday party. Dad's coming too, and Neil and his family. It will be the first time all of us have been together in the same country at the same time for many years. We'll be staying at an old mansion that my cousin and her husband have bought and turned into holiday-rental accommodation. We leave Edinburgh in convoy for the three-hour journey, and I drive with Dad.

When we arrive, on a beautiful, blue-sky afternoon, I do feel like a beer, but the moment is fleeting. I immerse myself in our family reunion and enjoy a weekend full of laughter. Previously, I would have marked this occasion by drinking my weight in wine; but being drunk can muddle some of the rich detail. This time, when I watch my aunty — who was widowed before I was born — slow-dance with her new partner, there are no beer goggles to obscure the sight, only my happy tears. The entire family, Scottish and English, bounces around the pub's dance floor, singing Proclaimers songs at the tops of our lungs, and I don't need wine to keep up. Later, as Mum clambers onto the bar — fuelled by malt whisky and an unwavering determination to cram as much fun into this lifetime as possible — I jump up with her, linking arms, partly to make sure she doesn't fall off and hasten the need for a second hip replacement, and partly because dancing on the bar with your 65-year-old mother just seems like something we should all do at least once in our lives. It's a reminder of the most important lesson I've learned in the last six months. When you take alcohol away, you have a choice: you either do the things you're scared to do completely sober, or you don't do them at all.

This weekend, I also tick off a goal I've been putting off for a very long time. For years, Mum has been asking me to sing for her. I've always made excuses. The last time she heard me sing publicly was at my high-school concert in my final year, when I was 18. Since then, due to a lack of confidence, the occasional drunken karaoke song is the closest I've got to live performance. When I stopped drinking, I ran out of excuses. So, every Monday night for the past few months, I've been brushing up on my skills by taking singing lessons, practising the song that Mum wants played at her funeral. 'Ain't Nobody's Business' is a sultry old jazz number that speaks of one woman's refusal to play by society's rules. It's an anthem for the way Mum lives her life, and the way she and Dad taught me to believe in myself and follow my own road, no matter what anyone says. If I wait until they're no longer around to hear me sing it, I'll regret it for the rest of my life.

So, in a pub full of people, mostly family, I get up and belt it out. I'm so nervous that it doesn't turn out to be the best performance I've ever given: I'm breathy, and my voice breaks a little when the emotion of the moment catches up with me. But I look at Mum, with tears streaking down her face, one hand over her mouth and the other raised in rhythmic salute to the music, and it's worth it. Few moments in life have given me greater satisfaction.

LEAVING DOESN'T GET any easier. Just when I'm wearing my Scottishness like a comfortable pair of old slippers, I'm off again. I'm lucky to have two incredible countries to call home, but this endless tug of war is no good for my heart.

I meet Fiona and her son, Jude, for a farewell coffee. I won't be here for his fifth birthday next month, so I give him his present now. His face, when he opens the gift, is a picture of delight. As I watch him, this good-natured wee boy with deep-blue eyes and a mop of blond hair, I'm in awe of my friend, who has raised two such wonderful children. She's not one for public displays of emotion; I'm the sappy, demonstrative one. I'll usually wait till we've had a few glasses of wine before I start gushing. But now, I say it anyway: I tell her those children are an absolute credit to her, and I'm proud of the family she's created and the success she's made of her life. We live on opposite sides of the world and I miss her terribly, but I've never seen her more contented — and that makes me happy.

When I get back to Melbourne, the first few weeks are hard. It's the same every time. I miss my parents, I miss my friends, and I miss my homeland. I vow, as I always do, that I will keep my accent. This time, without alcohol, which usually brings my Scottish enunciation charging back to the surface, it's even harder to hang on to. For a fortnight or so, I amuse my Melbourne friends by defiantly using Scots slang, and talking in a lilting brogue that's somewhere between an east-coast Billy Connolly and Begbie from *Trainspotting*, but it doesn't last. The Aussie inflections come back, my vowels lose their edge, and I'm once again fighting the urge to pound my chest and scream, 'Freedom!' when strangers hear my accent and ask if I'm American.

As I settle back into Melbourne life and reflect on the trip, I can't stop thinking about my past. Realising that I was drunk for much of my youth was confronting. I call Jon Currie and ask him to make arrangements for the brain scan and tests. That might be the only way to know if all that partying and waywardness has taken its toll. He tells me that it may take several months to get an appointment. That's okay — I'm curious, but I might need time to prepare for the results.

Many of the experiences I had in my teens and early adulthood were fun, and I wouldn't swap them; it was all part of growing up. But it makes me sad to think I relied on booze so much that even though I was bored with getting drunk, I felt socially paralysed without it. And it staggers me that the tempestuous relationship I developed with alcohol as a shy teenager carried on, unquestioned, for another 20 years. The myth that being boozed can help me to get a guy, boost my self-esteem, and make me more popular seems like lunacy after half a year without a drink.

A research project based on some of the *Hello Sunday Morning* blogs reveals that many young Australians see alcohol as a crucial element in their social life. As one blogger, Patrick, said: 'You celebrate you have a drink, you're depressed you have a drink, you finish an exam you have a drink, you finish work you have a drink, the footy's on you have a drink.'

Another observed: 'If my social circle were a pie chart, alcohol would account for about 90 per cent of it.'

But perhaps I'm not giving today's young people enough credit — maybe there are many 21st-century teens who are way too cool to believe that confidence is a liquid commodity. The Gen Y teen may be a more sophisticated beast than its grungy '90s predecessor. The only way to know is to ask them. My editor often speaks of her daughter Beth, a mature, savvy young woman who spent six months backpacking around Europe after she finished high school, and is now studying a Bachelor of Arts at the University of Melbourne.

The tales she brings home about boozy campus life have shocked even her usually unflappable mother. She talks of drinking games that start at ten in the morning and go on well into the night and the next morning. Getting pissed is such a part of uni life that Beth's already complaining she's over it. She's 19.

I decide that I must meet this girl. I've been knocking back booze longer than she's been alive, yet it's people like her who are in the eye of this binge-drinking storm. She might help me to understand whether today's teenagers and young adults really are bigger drinkers than previous generations, or if they're merely carrying on a way of life they inherited. And if they are huge drinkers, why do they place such importance on getting drunk?

I arrange to catch up with Beth and her friends Beck, who's also 19, and Emily, 20. We meet in a city beer garden, but surprisingly, even though I'm paying, they all order soft drinks. One has to work later, one is driving (as a P-plater, she can't have any alcohol in her system), and the third just doesn't feel like it. Well, these are hardly the boozed-up delinquents hooked on cheap grog the headlines would have us believe.

They tell me that they all started drinking in Year Nine, around the age of 15. One of their friends had parents who were relaxed about drinking, so they'd tell their folks they were going for a sleepover at her house and get smashed. By Year Ten, their own parents started buying them alcohol to take to parties. They didn't like the taste of beer, so pre-mixed spirits, or alcopops, were their favoured drinks. The right brand was important: Vodka Cruisers were cool; UDLs were for bogans. Beth would tell her parents that the six-pack would be shared with two friends. It wasn't. I realise that I'm about to learn more about my boss's daughter than my boss may know herself. I start to wonder if this was such a good idea.

Now that they're all of legal age, the girls say they still drink more at home than they do in clubs and bars. 'Very rarely do we go out and buy all our drinks out. We might have just a shot or one drink when you're at a club, but we'll pre-drink until we're at a comfortable level of drunkenness. Most young people of our age will avoid buying drinks out. It's so expensive,' Beth says.

Have they ever considered going out and not drinking? Emily, the only one in the group with a long-term boyfriend, says that she doesn't really drink to get drunk anymore, but she'll often have a drink just to have something in her hand. Beck says that she's been out a couple of times when she's the only one not drinking, and it wasn't fun. 'When you're sober, you just hate drunk people — they're really annoying. You'll be dancing or whatever and you just think, this is really boring. Why do we do this?'

I ask Beth how life would change if she didn't drink. 'Oh my God! I can't even imagine it. I'm very impressed that you're taking a year out,' she says, wide-eyed and smiling. 'One friend once said to us that when you're sober, you realise that going to a club is literally just all your friends standing in a circle bopping, and that's, like, all you're doing, but when you're drunk it's hilarious and it's the best time ever.' We both laugh. I don't think I've ever heard a more succinct description of my teenage years.

Beth continues, 'I definitely feel the pressure to drink when I go out. Like, not necessarily that people are making me drink, but I would feel like I wasn't going to have fun if I didn't drink. I've never gone out without drinking. I'm sure I could do it, but I have this mental thing where I think I'm not going to have fun. Drinking gives you a lot of confidence, and even if you're, like, making a massive fool of yourself, you don't feel like you are.'

Here's a witty, incredibly smart young woman who's more of a conversationalist than I could ever have hoped to be at that age, who thinks she's less than herself without alcohol. If she's already all of those things, what does she get from drinking?

'I think there's a certain thing where it's kind of cool to be drunk.

It doesn't necessarily mean you're going to be really embarrassing and everyone's going to be laughing at you. It's a cool element. They're the drunk person — "Oh, you were hilarious last night" — that kind of thing. There's an aspect of entertaining each other. You can get a reputation for being that big drinker who's always doing hilarious things when they're drunk, and that's sort of a positive in a way — until it's taken too far and you end up vomiting all over yourself, and then you're not so cool anymore.'

I can relate to that. I've struggled a bit with my identity since I stopped drinking. Who am I if not the loud girl at the party forcing everyone up to dance and making a goon of herself? People do gravitate towards the lively, drunk characters at parties, although admittedly sometimes they're laughing at them, not with them. But I've come to realise most of the things I don't do now that I might have when I was drunk would see me risking injury, unplanned pregnancy, vomiting, or a combination of all the above. The other fun stuff — dancing, meeting new people, singing off-key, cracking lame jokes, and behaving like a child with attention-deficit disorder — are still well within my remit of skills sober.

When they left school and started university, any doubts the girls may have had about drinking being the accepted and expected way of socialising were erased. The boozing began on day one of O (Orientation) Week. Beth talks about the University of Melbourne's annual induction camp for arts students as if it were a bacchanalian orgy. 'The basic aim of that camp is to be drunk the entire time, and have sex with as many people as you can while drunk. So we'd be in these huge dorms with bunks, and people would just be having sex, and everyone would be trashed. They have competitions to make you vomit. It's sort of sending the message that the only way you're going to meet people at uni is if you get smashed with them. You have to drink, otherwise you don't have a chance.'

The weekend camp is organised by former students, ensuring that the binge-drinking baton is passed down through the years. Drinking games are part of that tradition, with students competing in beer-sculling races, or encouraged to have 'one before ten' or 'ten before one': to down one drink before ten in the morning, when they're usually painfully hung-over, or have ten drinks before 1.00 p.m. All drinkers work in teams, and points are given for each completed task. Girls get extra points for taking their tops off. 'Everyone lost all their inhibitions. In the normal circumstance, people wouldn't, like, just take off all their clothes, but everyone suddenly felt comfortable to be completely naked. I didn't do it, but I sort of felt like I would because everyone's doing it and it seems fun,' Beth says. 'For a lot of people, that is an extremely attractive prospect — of just getting completely smashed the whole weekend. I think I was drunk from, like, the Friday night to Sunday afternoon. At night there's parties, and they do all sorts of competitions and dress-up stuff, and then in the day everyone just lies on the ground feeling disgusting. There's lots of throwing up, people passing out. It's very full-on.'

Beck, who goes to Monash University, says that things are similar there. 'They have a week during the semester called Green Week, which is supposed to be a celebration of beer. I'll be walking to and from lectures, and people are doing these obstacle courses involving drinking on the lawns. It looks really strange because other people are totally sober, just going to their classes, and there's this pile of people vomiting or doing stupid things.'

It sounds extreme, but students playing drinking games is hardly a new phenomenon. Green Week began at Monash in 1987. The following year, the student newspaper advertised the upcoming festivities with the line, 'If you can remember last year, you weren't really there.' The event promised 'five days of fun, frivolity, fornication and extremely high levels of intoxication', with free beer every day and sculling competitions.

Professor Rob Moodie, who was a student in the 1970s at the

University of Melbourne, where he is now chair of global health at
the Nossal Institute, told me that, when he was 21, he and fellow
undergraduates competed for the 'Bachelor of Imbibition'. This
marathon pub crawl around 24 watering holes saw contestants earn
qualifications for various drinks — a seven-ounce was a diploma, a
pot was a master's, and a glass of top-shelf was a PhD — in pursuit
of the ultimate prize, the bachelor, awarded for knocking back a
drink in every pub. The worse for wear would also finish with the
title 'BND' after their name — bloody near dead.

When young adults leave home and are thrust into a world of
freedom and new friends, which usually coincides with turning 18
and their first legal drink, they're going to party hard. But while
in Rob Moodie's day, drinking games were informal affairs thrown
together by groups of friends, these days pubs, university clubs, and
student unions are running organised drinking events. Some pubs
target the captains of university sports clubs, offering cheap drinks to
get them to bring teams to the venue. Sex is also used to sell booze.
To advertise student events, Pugg Mahones, an Irish bar in Carlton,
near the University of Melbourne, had on its website earlier this year
an image of a young woman in her bra, spreadeagled against some
beer kegs, while another woman, wearing a bra and jeans pushed
down to reveal her underwear, straddled and kissed her. The strapline
read, 'Because uni isn't all about study.' Beth says that those kind of
promotions aren't uncommon. The arts camp advertised its weekend
of fun with posters from *American Pie*, a teen movie about a group
of high-school students who pledge to lose their virginity before
graduation.

One concept that teenagers become familiar with from an early
age is getting drunk to pick up. Annual end-of-year schoolies events,
where students go wild at week-long parties in beach resorts across
Australia, have become famous for alcohol-fuelled sexual exploits.
A survey of 500 students at schoolies week on the Gold Coast in

2010 found that 60 per cent had more than ten drinks a night, and 'hooked up' (had intercourse or performed sexual acts) with a stranger at least once during the week. A quarter of boys and 4 per cent of girls also had sex with multiple partners. When the 17- to 19-year-olds were asked why they did it, many said it was the social norm: 'That's what you do when you're at schoolies.'

Having had a boyfriend for more than two years, Emily says that she found events such as schoolies and O Week a challenge. 'It wasn't just that I didn't want to sleep around, or even the kissing. It's that culture of, everyone's getting a bit loose, we're at a concert, and all of my friends around me are turning around and making out with the guys they're dancing with, whereas I didn't want a guy to touch me, I was pushing them away. Going to clubs, it's fun to drink, and I still enjoy the dancing, but the whole interaction with the opposite sex is fuelled by this sex thing coming into it. I don't always feel comfortable going out because guys do touch you and grind up against you. You can't just casually chat with guys because a lot of the time their end goal is to ask you if you want to come back to their house.'

Beth agrees that alcohol is a 'huge part' of interacting with the opposite sex, and says that it helps her to talk to guys. At high-school parties, 'hooking up' — by which they mean kissing — was often the sole point of the evening, but now it's less important. None of them have hooked up with a new guy sober. 'If you're drunk and you're really confident and you're talking to everyone and you're being loud, I think guys find that attractive — that confidence, although it's artificial. If you're the centre of attention, guys like that,' Beth says.

The pressure to drink doesn't just come from their schooling experiences. Both Beth and Emily have worked in office jobs in the finance industry, where they saw an entrenched binge-drinking culture, a pattern of behaviour every Friday night, which was often led by colleagues much older than them. Emily was taunted for months after she left a boozy office Christmas party early. 'I'm still confident in my choices, and I try to not be affected by people teasing me about not drinking with them, but it still affects me. My cool factor is apparently based on how late I can stay out and how much I drink,' she says.

For Beth, it was eye-opening. 'I was really surprised that the [office] drinking culture is just as strong as uni drinking culture. And it didn't really matter what age you were — everyone wanted to do it. It highlighted that it's everybody, it's Australia. The media concentrates on youth, but everyone else is doing it too.'

The statistics back Beth's theory up. Baby boomers may shake their heads at the binge-drinking habits of their kids and grandkids, but it may well be that young people have inherited unhealthy drinking patterns from older generations. Figures from the Australian Institute of Health and Welfare's 2010 National Drug Strategy Household Survey show that older Australians are much more likely to drink every day than their children are. Ten per cent of people in their fifties drink daily, rising to 13 per cent of those in their sixties, and 15 per cent of people aged 70 or older. That compares to just 2 per cent of 20-somethings, about 1 per cent of teenagers, and an average of 8 per cent across all age groups. And while young people are drinking to excess in greater numbers than older people, their elders are not far behind. The survey found that 21 per cent of those in their fifties regularly drink in a way that puts them at risk of long-term health problems, compared to 27 per cent of 20-somethings and 32 per cent of 18- to 19-year-olds.

While all the focus is on binge drinking among younger generations, alcohol experts say that there are huge problems ahead for their parents and grandparents. As Professor Steve Allsop, director of the National Drug Research Institute, told me during my 'Alcohol Timebomb' series: 'Even if nothing changes, we're going to have a substantial increase over the next 20 years of older people who are drinking at levels that cause harm to themselves and potentially to others. And it may be that things get worse rather than better because if the baby boomers take their drinking habits into older age, that's going to be a real problem.'

Drinking may be an integral part of Beth's world, but, despite the pub crawls and the wasted weekends, she's realised that getting pissed is not what makes her popular. 'Most of the good friends I've made at uni, I've made in lectures and tutes because when you're drunk the whole time, you don't really make friends. You get to know people, but you don't learn about each other — you're just drunk together. People don't realise how dependent they become on alcohol. I sometimes take a step back and think, oh my God, I'm so dependent, I've got to try and go out without drinking that much.'

As I've discovered at 35, it's hard to walk a different path from your friends. At 19, it's got to be near impossible. Alcohol experts say that, to change the culture, we need to show young people that not drinking is just as valued by society as getting drunk. The rise of social media has made that more challenging. In a study conducted by Brad Ridout from the University of Sydney, boozy Facebook profiles were found to be creating a social contagion effect, normalising binge drinking and encouraging more young people to get pissed. The study of 163 university students aged 17 to 24 found that those who saw alcohol as a strong part of their online identity were likely to drink more to keep up their party-animal image. They were also more likely to have blackouts, get into fights, or have sexual encounters they later regretted. A recent British study found that the average Facebook user is drunk or drinking in 76 per cent of pictures they post on the site. I suspect that if I did an analysis of my own Facebook page, I'd reach a similar conclusion.

In research conducted by Dr Nicholas Carah from the University of Queensland, which used young *Hello Sunday Morning* participants as subjects, bloggers described Facebook as an 'archive for wild nights out', where the dominant portrayal of drinking is glorified, and the drinking itself is made to seem excessive. One described the status-update cycle on Facebook as 'Who's going out?' in the evening, and in the morning, 'I'm so hung-over — why did I go out?' Rather than posting pictures of academic achievements, young people talk up their drunken antics, and are praised for it. The sicker you feel the next morning, the more kudos you get.

When blogger Andrew joined *Hello Sunday Morning*, he went through his Facebook photos and deleted all the ones in which he was drunk or had a drink in his hand. 'I ended up deleting, like, two-thirds of my photos ... People take their cameras round because ... that's the way they know what happened last night.'

Beth says that she has no plans to stop drinking. She's by no means a massive drinker, in comparison to some her age: on an average night out, she'll have six or seven drinks. Unlike some of her friends, she hasn't mastered the 'strat vom' (strategic vomit), where you stick your fingers down your throat and make yourself sick so that you can keep drinking; when she drinks too much, that's the end of her night. She admits that when her mum told her about me still getting drunk on the weekends, she was surprised. But after thinking about it for a while, it didn't seem so weird. 'I was like, well, I enjoy drinking and I enjoy getting drunk, so I don't actually know what would happen to me to make me stop doing it.'

The alcohol campaigns warning young people about the perils of binge drinking miss the mark with these girls — they don't relate to images of kids being arrested or beaten up. What might sway them is an advert highlighting the health hazards of too much booze: they know that it's bad for their livers, but that's where their knowledge ends. The kind of statistics that Craig Sinclair from the Cancer Council highlighted, about the risk of breast cancer, might be enough to get their attention. 'You're not quite aware what you're doing to your body when you're drinking in excess, but with smoking, the advertising about that, and the stigma, was so strong that I knew I didn't want to be a smoker,' Beth says. 'But I didn't feel the same thing for alcohol. It's such an inherent part of Australian culture. If there were adverts that really showed you what you're actually doing to yourself when you're drinking, you might stop and think. That's probably what smoking was like 50 years ago.'

After I leave Beth and her friends, I think about their experiences and conclude they're not dissimilar to mine at that age. They're probably not drinking any more than I did, and I must confess to being a fan of the old 'strat vom' in my early twenties, although we didn't have cool shorthand for it back then — it was just a self-induced drunken spew. The big difference is how much more insight they have into the drinking culture they inhabit. They're aware that using booze as a social crutch is not a great long-term strategy. They know that it's probably bad for their health. Yet they still drink regularly. Their peers and their community expect it of them; and when they try to opt out, they feel shunned. If these switched-on young women think that it's more acceptable to binge drink than it is to drink moderately or to abstain, then this isn't just a youth problem. They live in a community that exalts drinking as the cornerstone of all social interaction: their bosses tell them that not having Friday knock-off drinks is un-Australian; their parents buy them booze and teach them that a glass of wine is how to unwind after a tough day; and their music festivals are sponsored by alcohol companies, and headlined by multi-millionaires who sing songs about getting wasted. Can we really expect them to drink moderately in this environment?

As I reach seven months of sobriety, this point is underscored tragically when Amy Winehouse is found dead in her London flat. The divinely talented 27-year-old singer, who battled addiction and penned a defiant hit about resisting rehab, literally drank herself to an early grave — vodka bottles were found next to her body. Within hours, wailing fans were getting pissed outside her home, sobbing and belting out her songs. They created a shrine using, along with flowers and cards, beer cans, wine glasses, and bottles of vodka and gin. It seems that even if it kills you, alcohol's cool.

August

LAST NIGHT, FOR the first time since I stopped drinking, I didn't feel like the odd one out. At a reunion dinner with friends from my *Age* traineeship of five years ago, the non-drinkers were equal in numbers to the drinkers. Of the eight of us, two were pregnant, one doesn't drink, and then there was me, the social animal of our year — who, on our induction trip to Sydney, was one of the last to go to bed, after persuading everyone to have one more for the road and join me in a rendition of 'Flower of Scotland' — now sensible and sober. Three of them have since left *The Age*, and one works in our Canberra bureau, so we rarely get to catch up as a group.

It was a fun evening, with lively conversation, fond memories, and, for once, a mocktail list that was both interesting and reasonably priced. But as we spilled out onto the street around 11 o'clock, I was reminded of why I rarely venture into the city after 9.00 p.m. Young guys clutching cans of bourbon and Coke were hollering to their mates and jumping into the road, trying to hail cabs; girls in skimpy dresses smoked cigarettes and screamed out incoherently against the backdrop of an ambulance siren. We flagged down a cab and adopted a women-and-children-first policy, sending our pregnant friends home before the rest of the group.

As we drove out of the city, it seemed that Melbourne was one heaving mass of drunkenness. The staff that work in these late-night venues must have balls of steel.

I used to be one of them — I spent more than ten years working in bars. From my first job at 18, in Dad's golf club, to an Irish pub in Christchurch, New Zealand, and a homely boozer in Melbourne, bar work taught me patience, diplomacy, and people skills. And it toughened me up. I learned pretty quickly how to escape the advances of drunk businessmen and how to defuse a fight before it started. Copping verbal abuse, wiping up spew, and being hit on by cavemen was just part of the job.

For the most part, I loved it. And I was good at it. At the Jekyll & Hyde in Edinburgh's New Town — a horror-themed pub, where the toilets were hidden behind a false bookcase and staff donned lab coats to sell cocktail-filled test tubes, before performing the Time Warp en masse at last orders — I learned to pour three pints at once, ensuring that a queue of thirsty punters were served speedily enough to avoid a riot. It was a good laugh. I made lifelong friends and met some fascinating customers.

Bar work even led to my first big break in journalism. Among the regulars at Champagne Charlies, a small, city-centre Edinburgh bar popular with suits, was a group of guys from Scotland's then highest-selling newspaper, *The Daily Record*. I was a first-year journalism student who used to practice her shorthand on cigarette breaks. I hassled the boys about work experience every time they came into the pub. I had something they wanted: beer. They had something I wanted: access to a national newspaper. It seemed a fair swap. I got my work-experience placement and, just over a year after finishing my degree, via stints at a local paper and a press agency, these pub regulars became my colleagues when I landed a job at the *Record*.

But bar work is for the young and nimble. Being on your feet for nine hours and knocking off at 3.00 a.m. loses its appeal when your bones are creaking and you're ready for a nana nap by ten o'clock. Your threshold for tolerating drunken idiots also drops. But more than anything, it gets harder to keep up with the lifestyle. Boozy lock-ins were common in six of the seven pubs and clubs I worked in. Even if you worked a day shift, you'd knock off, sit on the other side of the bar with your workmates, and pour your wages back into the till.

There's a collegial atmosphere when you're part of an unburdened workforce of students and backpackers in their twenties. On busy shifts, bar work can feel like trench warfare: it's you and your mates behind the barricades, against the snarling hordes on the other side. Nothing speeds up the bonding process quite like an inebriated halfwit trying to feel up one of your new friends as she clears tables. When I was a backpacker in Christchurch, my workmates at The Bog Irish Bar became my surrogate family. We worked hard and played harder. It was one of the happiest times of my life, although much of it is a blur. Looking back at travel diaries, it seems that I drank for more than 300 of the 365 days I spent in New Zealand. My travelling buddy Sharon, who I met working at Jekyll & Hyde, got a job in an office and wasn't far behind me, but I think working in a pub definitely meant that I drank more than she did.

I'm not surprised to learn that a 2007 study out of Britain's Office for National Statistics found that bar staff in England and Wales were twice as likely to die from alcohol-related problems as the general population. Researchers speculated that the high risk levels might be related to social pressure to drink at work, lack of supervision, separation from family members, and the recruitment of people who were already heavy drinkers. I think about the bars I've worked in, where young backpackers are thousands of kilometres away from their parents, and colleagues share the night's horror stories over knock-off drinks. It's not difficult to see how an unhealthy pattern might develop. Full-time bar work makes it easy to fall into a habit of daily drinking.

It has been five years since I pulled beers when I started my only bar job in Melbourne. I'd been struggling to get full-time work in journalism since moving from Scotland, and, even though I was freelancing for *The Age*, it wasn't enough to pay the rent — so I found myself returning to the only other trade I knew. At 29, I wasn't overly enthused by the prospect of getting back behind the bar. I was too old to hack the pace in nightclubs and late-night bars, so I found a pub that kept civilised hours. The Rose Hotel in Fitzroy is an old-school, no-frills pub, where the walls are adorned with pictures of footy legends, and the locals keep their personalised stubby holders behind the bar. The decor, which looks like it's hardly changed since the pub was opened in 1861, has a cosy, lounge-room feel. Just two streets back from the Brunswick Street party precinct, this homely boozer is a rarity in a suburb that's become so gentrified, the blue-collar workers who built it have been largely priced out of the area. There's trivia on Monday, and a meat-tray raffle every Friday night; it's a country pub in the middle of the inner city.

The alcohol and hospitality industries cop a lot of flak for fuelling Australia's binge-drinking problem, but it's not all aircraft hangar–sized nightclubs and 24-hour bargain-basement bottle shops. There are lots of places like The Rose, where people feel connected to their neighbours. In country towns, communities are built around the pub, with social events, sports clubs, and fundraisers often organised through the local watering hole. In the city, it's less common; bars can be cold and uninviting, their trade and staff transient. That's why I fell in love with The Rose. It's a pub with a soul. Each year they stage a street party to raise funds for the local primary school. The bar's also part of a pub cricket league, involving 14 Fitzroy establishments that play off before an end-of-season 'Super Sunday' event, which attracts hundreds of people and brings in cash for local charities.

My first shift was a baptism of fire: a wake for the former owner, a formidable woman who had run the pub, with her husband, for 13 years, before selling up in 2001, when my former boss, Tony, and his wife, George, took over. Hundreds of people had gone to the funeral, far more than the small chapel could cater for. Many came back to The Rose afterwards, to continue the celebration of their former publican's life. They raised their glasses to her good humour and generosity, and played the Hawthorn club song again and again for a woman who lived for footy and had become a substitute mother to many of the locals. Laconic men with callused hands and sun-blasted skin shed tears openly. Then there was laughter, as they remembered her inability to suffer fools. I realised very quickly that this was more than a pub — it was a community. For me, thousands of kilometres away from my family, and after four years without a stable job to which to anchor myself, working at The Rose was the first time Melbourne felt like home.

I go back to the pub to speak to Tony, and to my friend Brigitte, a Rose regular I met over the bar and went on an overseas holiday with a few years back. When I walk in, there's Brian the plumber sitting on his usual stool, drinking James Squire. When he leaves, he gives Tony a wave and lays his empty pot glass on its side on the bar, as he always does. Andy, another plumber and the former social club president, embraces me warmly. As usual, he's drinking his VB in a stubby holder, with a copper handle he made himself. It's 5.30 on a Thursday evening, and the bar is filled with the usual eclectic mix of blue-collar workers, office staff, old blokes and young blokes, families, hipsters, goths, and students.

Tony greets me with his usual 'Jilly!', and we hug as I remind him that I'm his favourite barmaid. He may or may not have uttered these words during knock-off drinks one night, but I turned it into indisputable fact and never let him forget it. He can't quite believe I've gone this long without drinking. When he took me on in 2005, I was one of the few people who drank cider; he used to joke that the pub went through more Strongbow in the months after he hired me than they had in the previous year.

The three of us sit down in the dining room, and I ask Tony what the pub means to his regulars. He tells me it's a place of safety and familiarity. He holds, behind the bar, many sets of house keys, left in his care by locals in case they lock themselves out. 'It's what makes the pub good for me and what makes it different from all the other pubs. It's got that human touch to it, and it's connected. It keeps you very earthed. It makes you realise it's not just about making money,' he says.

One of my favourite Rose regulars was an old bloke called Jack, known to the locals as 'the old diamond'. Most weekdays, this then 89-year-old former boxer would drive his Mazda 323 to the pub, park himself at the bar, and do the crossword while drinking a beer. He'd come in at about 11.30 a.m. and stay for a couple of hours. We'd chat about his life, football, and the weather. He'd crack jokes at Tony's expense, and call me 'lass' in a grandfatherly way. Sometimes he'd pick up his groceries on the way to the pub, and I'd pop his lamb's brains in the fridge, on top of the Coopers Green, to keep them cool. Now, at 95, he lives in a nursing home. He no longer drives. But he still comes to the pub by taxi. His family were wary about his regular visits as he grew older, worried for his health. Tony sat down with them recently and worked it out. 'I said to them, "If he doesn't come here, he will last a couple of months and he'll die because all he lives for is to come here." He's got no friends at the home, but he's got a lot of friends here. He walks in, he gets seated, he gets his glasses handed to him, he gets the newspaper given to him, he gets his beer, he's got his own chair. So for someone like him, coming to the pub is the difference between life and death. We came up with a compromise: we agreed to take him from heavy beer to light beer, and his family would leave his taxi money behind the bar so we can pay the driver.'

Jack comes in three days a week and drinks two or three pots of light beer. There's no money in customers like him. But for Tony, these are the punters that make coming to work worthwhile. 'The pub's been good to us. We've met so many good people through here. It's been fantastic in that sense, and that's the biggest spin-off for us. There would be a huge hole if this pub went. Just that meeting place, that connection. I just think of our friends — I have no idea where they would go.'

There's no doubt that The Rose is a second home for many regulars. I could walk in there any day of the week and the same groups of drinkers would be standing in their usual spot at the bar, or at their favourite table, just as they did six years ago when I was pouring their beers. That familiarity is comforting, but I remember wondering back then if it was more than that for some of the locals. The men who would spend five, six, seven, or more hours a day, every day, in the pub couldn't be spending much time with their wives and kids. When they'd try to leave, they'd be badgered by their mates to have one more for the road. For some, a few beers down the local was more than a ritual; it was a problem.

The Rose sits just a block away from the controversial 'Cheese Grater' complex — an eight-storey apartment block that was completed in 2010, despite years of legal wrangling and more than 550 objections from local residents and businesses, who argued that it would ruin the character of the area. As more apartment buildings spring up, locals worry that these high-density dwellings will further erode Fitzroy's community feel. Tony laughs when he tells me it may be the pub that stops this from happening. 'It's funny, with the Cheese Grater and a few of the other high-rise apartment blocks that have gone up, they don't socialise at all in those blocks. They all just go in, get in the lifts, in their front door, and they don't see each other. Then they come here to the pub, and they get talking to people and they go, "Oh, you live in the same block as me. We're two doors from each other," or, "We're on the same floor." It becomes a real hub of your community, where people actually meet each other and their neighbours more than they do in their own home.'

Tony says his priority as a publican is to ensure that no-one comes to harm, even after they leave the premises. 'They're all grown-ups, and I'm not there to be their parent and tell them what they can and can't do because quite often you're doing more harm by just throwing them out anyway. They'll just go off and stagger somewhere else. For some people, you're better off keeping them here where you can keep an eye on them. I've walked people home from here, I've driven people home, I've had people walk off from here and I've had to go and find them.'

I think I only refused to serve a customer on a handful of occasions during my six-month stint at The Rose. With a pub full of regulars, it was hard to say no, even when you knew they'd had too much. But how much is too much? Alcohol-related violence across Melbourne has led to a crackdown on irresponsible service. Bar owners and individual staff members are liable for big fines for serving intoxicated patrons. The liquor licensing department has stepped up its random checks. But the definition of intoxication is open to interpretation. To the letter of the law, it's hard to see how Tony can legally serve anyone.

According to the Victorian liquor licensing department's guide on how to spot a drunk person, the signs of intoxication are many and varied. There are the no-brainers: violent behaviour, vomiting, falling over, or sleeping at the bar. But then there are more subtle changes in behaviour: becoming argumentative, annoying other patrons and staff, using offensive language, or displaying inappropriate sexual behaviour. Physical signs include spilling drinks, glassy eyes and lack of focus, swaying and staggering, and bumping into furniture. Finally, you might notice changes in alertness: rambling conversation, loss of train of thought, and difficulty in paying attention. They're helpful tips, but if I'd cut off every sleazy windbag who used foul language, talked shit, and knocked a drink over on the way to the toilet, my bar-wench career would have been over very quickly. The guidelines point out that this list is by no means exhaustive, and does not necessarily give conclusive evidence of intoxication, but they do expect a lot from staff, who are probably on minimum wage and face landing their boss with fines of up to $14,000 if they get it wrong.

'Prior to refusing service on the basis that a person is intoxicated, you must be able to rule out various medical conditions and disabilities that cause symptoms similar to intoxication. For example, possible illness, injury, or medical conditions such as brain trauma, hypoglycaemia, or pneumonia,' the guidelines advise. So on a Saturday night when it's three-deep at the bar, the music's pumping, and they can't hear their own voice above the cackles of a wayward hen's party, the bartender is expected to weigh up symptoms and make a diagnosis before deciding if the slurring punter in front of them has had one too many shandies or is in fact a stroke victim? It seems like a lot to ask. In my experience in busy venues, particularly in clubs and late-night bars, there's very little time to make an assessment of the customer's ability to handle another drink. It's a production line: the faster you can get the drinks out, the more people you can serve, and the easier your night will be.

At small, family-friendly pubs like The Rose, it's simpler to spot someone who's wasted. And a lot of the time, you'll know them. You'll know if they're a bit pissed, but harmless. You'll know how to take the heat out of the situation, and make them laugh when they get argumentative. And if things do get out of hand, the other regulars will help you out.

Tony has a zero-tolerance policy on violence and aggression in his pub. It's a standpoint the locals fully support. Although the incidence of violence is low — I can remember only one punch being thrown in all the time I worked at The Rose, and that was between two university mates arguing about whether the death penalty was barbaric — if something kicks off, it will quickly be shut down by the regulars. 'We just don't tolerate it,' Brigitte says. 'We'll tell them it's not on, to take it elsewhere. You look at your bar staff too, and your management. Do you have bar staff who are invested in the pub and are friends with the people over the bar, who have a relationship with those people? Or are they just there to look good? You can defuse so many situations if you actually have a relationship with the people you're serving.'

Having staff and clientele who feel a connection with the pub may explain why The Rose very rarely attracts trouble, despite being just a few hundred metres from Brunswick Street, where there's always a strong police presence and most of the bars have bouncers on the door. Brigitte, who has lived just off Brunswick Street for five years, has noticed a change recently. 'In our place it's normally very quiet, with the way the building's facing, but the last six to 12 months, the amount of fights we've heard, the amount of bottles being thrown ... We even heard a gunshot about three or four months ago, which I've never heard before. It just seems to be getting worse and worse.'

There's no one answer to explain this shift in behaviour, but the increasing availability of booze surely plays a part. The liberalisation of alcohol laws in Victoria in the late 1980s and 1990s led to an avalanche of new liquor licences. In 2011, there are more than 19,000 outlets selling booze — a 77 per cent increase on 2000. Preventative Health Taskforce chair Rob Moodie maintains that Victoria has gone from the 'wowser state' to the 'wet and sloshed state'. Over the same period, alcohol-related ambulance callouts increased by 258 per cent, hospitalisations went up by 87 per cent, assaults by 49 per cent, and family violence incidents in which alcohol was a contributing factor doubled. A few years ago, when my Fitzroy gym started selling beer and my hairdressing salon offered me free champagne with my blow-wave, I remember thinking that there aren't many places left where you can't get a drink in this town.

As I say my goodbyes to Tony and Brigitte, I think about the contrast between the convivial atmosphere of The Rose and that of the neighbouring Brunswick Street. It's hard to believe that the two co-exist in such close proximity. I've seen the aggression — when you're living in the inner city, it's hard to avoid. I stopped drinking in Brunswick Street years ago, partly because I moved further out, but also because the friendly village feel that used to make it so appealing has all but gone. The troubles of the city seem to be creeping further north, enveloping our bar and cafe strips in simmering tension. Being sober makes it even more noticeable. Driving home through Fitzroy one night recently, the atmosphere on the street was charged and hostile. Stopped at the traffic lights, watching drinkers bouncing around erratically like characters in a video game, I couldn't wait to get out of there.

A lot of the trouble seems to start in queues, as drinkers lose patience with lining up to get into crowded venues. Police say that the smoking ban inside pubs has exacerbated the problem: more people hanging around outside bars and clubs to have a ciggie leads to more altercations with passing punters. It's a trend the police are trying to combat: a 6 per cent increase in assaults in 2010 in the City of Yarra — which takes in the popular inner-city drinking areas of Fitzroy, Collingwood, and Richmond — led to a crackdown on antisocial behaviour. Pissed punters caught damaging cars and shops, getting into fights, drinking on the street, or being drunk and disorderly were arrested, handed on-the-spot fines, or banned from the area for 24 hours. The operation was deemed a success. Still, once a suburb is sprawling with cops, you can't help thinking that some of its charm has been lost.

What's interesting about this rise in aggression is that it's not just blokes picking fights. I've seen women throw punches; I've watched them get kicked out of pubs for abusing bar staff. The rise of a phenomenon described somewhat unimaginatively as 'ladette culture' means that sculling drinks, getting wasted in public, and being cheered on by your mates for drunken bad behaviour is no longer left to the boys. While men are still binge drinking at higher rates than women, the girls are catching up, as rates for blokes are slowing, or, in some age groups, declining. Between 2002 and 2009, the proportion of Victorian women aged 16 to 24 who had knocked back 20 drinks in one sitting on at least one occasion in the previous year jumped from 15 per cent to 32 per cent. Across all ages, the number of Victorian women charged with alcohol-related family-violence offences jumped from 27 per year in 2000–01 to 147 in 2009–10, while over the same period, their rate of emergency-department presentations for intoxication increased at more than twice the rate of men, leaping from 785 a year, to 1874. Researchers talk of an emerging 'badge of honour' mentality, where some young women celebrate extreme drunkenness, aggression, and violence as signs that they're keeping up with the boys. It's good that the pub trade has moved past the days where the only women allowed in bars were the ones pouring the beer, but it's a sad indictment on our culture that the quest for sexual equality means some young women feel compelled to drink so much they end up in hospital, or become so aggressive they're arrested for getting into fights or, more worryingly, as police are increasingly reporting, for glassing incidents.

I can honestly say that, while being drunk has contributed to some silly arguments with friends and the occasional spat with workmates, I've never found myself so plastered that I feel the urge to shove glassware in someone's face. But as a former bartender, I wonder how much I've contributed to the culture of antisocial drinking we're now witnessing. In my decade of bar work across three countries, I regularly served pissed people. I encouraged excessive drinking through ridiculously cheap happy-hour promotions and, in one pub, offered free drinks to anyone who could down a yard of ale. I served Guinness and Jameson to thirsty Irishmen at 7.00 a.m. on St Patrick's Day, and lined up shots on the bar for fresh-faced customers without checking their IDs. On both sides of the bar, I have been irresponsible.

But public-health experts argue that the problem goes beyond the actions of the bartender or the personal responsibility of the drinker. They blame the alcohol industry as a whole. These days, bottle-shop booze is so cheap that many people are drunk before they leave the house. Just like Beth and her friends, who 'pre-drink until [they're] at a comfortable level of drunkenness', many young people are well on their way to being smashed by the time they head into Melbourne's entertainment precincts. The health lobby claims that systemic discounting, in tandem with aggressive marketing and a proliferation of liquor licences, have left our streets awash with booze. Rob Moodie describes this discounting as the 'Bunningsisation of alcohol', where a bottle of wine can be sold for less than $3 in massive cut-price warehouses, and punters are encouraged to buy in bulk and load up shopping trolleys with grog. A 2009 analysis found that large liquor barns were responsible for 70 per cent of all Australian alcohol advertising, up from 30 per cent in 1989. Adverts for boutique stores fell from 29 per cent to just 5 per cent.

It probably doesn't help that Australia's leading supermarket chains control half of the country's liquor supply. Woolworths, which owns Dan Murphy's and BWS, and Coles, which owns Liquorland, First Choice, and Vintage Cellars, leverage their duopoly regularly to undercut competitors, using heavily discounted alcohol as a loss leader. In March 2011, Foster's was forced to withhold the supply of key brands, including VB and Carlton Draught, when it learned that the supermarket giants were planning to sell them for $28 a slab, well below cost. The brewer said the discounting undermined their brands.

Some of my friends have begged me to stop giving health experts a platform to condemn cheap, all-night booze as an inherently bad thing. They have read my stories about a blitz on late-night bottle shops, or calls for an end to discounting, and sent me half-joking text messages asking what I have against affordable, readily available grog. But while slashing the price of booze might be a boon for the average drinker, it's usually the community's most vulnerable who suffer. According to the World Health Organization, underage and heavy drinkers are the groups most likely to drink excessively when booze is cheap. Nowhere is that more apparent than in Australia's Indigenous communities, where alcohol abuse has ravaged towns, and the rate of drinking-related deaths is twice that of the general population, through chronic disease, accidents, violence, and suicide. In June 2011, in response to alcohol-fuelled violence in Alice Springs and to criticisms that its cheap booze was contributing to the problem, Coles announced that, from 1 July, it would stop selling two-litre casks of wine — a product that sold for less than 50 cents a standard drink. A minimum price of $8 was brought in for bottles of wine. Woolworths quickly followed suit. The retail giants ruled out extending the policy to the rest of Australia, but there may be changes ahead: the federal government has asked its National Preventive Health Agency to investigate the merits of a national floor price for alcohol, similar to the one being introduced in Scotland.

It's not just Indigenous communities that are hit hard by heavily discounted booze. A few years back, I reported that price wars had become so fierce, some smaller bottle shops were offering public-housing tenants credit and free home delivery, in a bid to compete with the big chains. Some customers on pensions had racked up massive debts and were being hounded by loan sharks. Research by Turning Point and VicHealth shows that disadvantaged areas are flooded with bottle shops, with up to six times as many outlets as wealthier neighbourhoods. Studies have consistently shown that areas with a high number of bottle shops have greater rates of chronic disease, risky drinking, assaults, and domestic violence. It raises the question: is the alcohol industry deliberately targeting poor people?

In 2007, I found out what happens when a local community tries to fight back against the proliferation of cheap grog. Preston, a traditionally working-class suburb in Melbourne's inner north, is part of the City of Darebin — a council area with the second-highest rate of alcohol-related deaths in Melbourne. The suburb was experiencing unprecedented levels of underage drinking, with kids buying cheap booze, and running amok in parks and at parties. Alcohol-related assaults, criminal damage, domestic violence, and health problems were also climbing rapidly. Police said that much of the trouble was originating near bottle shops, where drinking was much harder to control than in licensed venues. When an application for a small wine store was lodged with the liquor-licensing department, police and council lodged a joint objection, on the grounds that it would harm the community by encouraging more alcohol abuse. There were already 65 places in Preston to buy alcohol, including 11 bottle shops. That, they argued, was more than enough. In a landmark legal case, Victoria's then director of liquor licensing, Sue Maclellan, upheld the objection. It was the first time that a licence had been turned down on the grounds of social harm. Health experts lauded it as a major win in the fight to turn around our alcohol culture.

But the victory was short-lived. Six weeks later, Maclellan granted a licence for a Dan Murphy's superstore in Preston. The council and police objected, on the same basis as their previous complaint. Maclellan dismissed it. As Geoff Munro, a long-time alcohol campaigner from the Australian Drug Foundation, told me at the time, 'It's hard to understand the logic of granting a licence to a mega-discount liquor store when a smaller discount liquor store was rejected on the grounds that it might exacerbate existing alcohol harms. It's just extraordinary. It's time we had a balanced liquor-licensing law that took account of people's health and not just the economic interests of liquor merchants.'

The following week, community frustration turned to fury when I discovered that the proposed Dan Murphy's store was to be less than 200 metres from a Salvation Army rehabilitation facility. Women battling alcoholism would have a perfect view of the liquor giant from their bedroom windows.

To this day, I've not received an answer from Maclellan about the inconsistency of her decisions. There's no suggestion that she did anything improper or was unduly influenced by the might of Dan Murphy's, but there's no doubt that the liquor giant has access to far greater legal resources than any small business fighting a licensing decision. The owner of the family-run chain of wine stores who had his licence application refused told me, 'It all boils down to one thing: the big get bigger and the small get smaller. There's no way any independent will ever beat the chains.' The result of this stranglehold on competition is ever-cheaper alcohol.

Since I stopped drinking, I've begun to notice just how insidious this proliferation of cut-price booze has become. Much like dieters who see chocolate cake and pizza everywhere they look, I feel as if I'm under siege from dirt-cheap grog. And the more you buy, the cheaper it is. The full-page, and often double-page, adverts in the national press are so ubiquitous that I can't read my own paper without being bombarded by beer. I may have left bar work behind, but it seems that the alcohol industry is still keeping me in a job.

I'M HAVING LUNCH with a man who's heard it all before. As a senior alcohol-industry executive, he's grown accustomed to being called names; he's had to develop a Teflon exterior. Health experts have accused his industry of being disease vectors, of trying to lure children into a lifetime of binge drinking, and of putting profits ahead of people. He stopped getting angry a long time ago. Now, he just seems tired.

We meet in one of Melbourne's high-end restaurants — his choice, and on his tab. It's a shame that I can't join him in a glass of wine; the list of offerings is exquisite. Plus, I quite like the idea of getting sozzled with a corporate bigwig, whiling away the afternoon quaffing Moët & Chandon and Rémy Martin, safe in the knowledge that the bill is being picked up by the very industry charged with transforming me, and countless others, into binge-drinking reprobates. But my decadent fantasy will have to wait for another day. I order mineral water.

I've debated this man many times. He's engaging and whip-smart. His response to claims against the industry is always considered and fair. He often shows a healthy degree of wariness in answering my questions, but today he seems more apprehensive than usual. In fact, he tells me that he does not want to be named in my book.

I start by asking him what he thought when he read the article about my history of binge drinking. He says he was surprised that someone who, he had presumed from my reporting, had a dim view of alcohol abuse would drink so much. 'It's a bit like a police reporter being caught shoplifting,' he says. I laugh, and he seems to relax a bit. 'I wouldn't have said it changed the credibility of what you wrote because you've always been reasonably fair.'

It's a generous concession from a man whose industry I have repeatedly hammered in the pages of *The Age* and *The Sunday Age*. While he's in such a mood, I ask him to be completely frank. I know that he's paid to represent the alcohol industry's best interests, but just quietly, there must be times when he thinks, hang on, maybe my industry does fuel harmful drinking?

He doesn't hesitate. 'I don't think it does now, and I don't think it has done ever. The public-health lobby, like so many social-justice groups, see the industry as vastly more powerful and controlling than it actually is. We're actually led by our customers far more than us leading them. We might bring out a new product, and if people like it, well, that's great; it's not some sort of Machiavellian plan to find new ways that people can drink more and more. We see what people want and we provide it for them. It's not like we have magical means of saying, "Here, everyone drink more and drink quicker."'

But drinking more we are. If market forces have played no part in our current binge-drinking culture, how did we get here? He puts it down to rapid social changes. Young people are reaching independence at an earlier age, and are having a longer period of freedom before taking on 'marriage, mortgage, and maternity'. This, along with a long economic boom in which jobs have been fairly easy to come by, has made it a golden time for young Australians. 'When people are confident about their jobs and things are going well, they celebrate,' he says. But he also blames a 'me culture', where the rise of bigger cities means that people can be more anonymous, and social norms have moved from self-restraint to excess. In essence, public standards have slipped; drunkenness and drunken notoriety are now seen as socially acceptable.

I suggest, respectfully, that the industry, culpable or not, must be happy with a society where excessive drinking is the norm. Isn't the bottom line to increase sales? He disagrees. 'We're led by our consumers. If our consumers want to drink less, well, we'll sell them less, because we'd have no option and we'd just have to cope with that change, which would happen over a long period of time. The industry will adapt. We will sell them better. We will move them on to more heavily branded items, higher quality products, and at higher prices. If everybody was limited to having half a bottle of wine a week, people wouldn't spend that much less on wine, but they'd be drinking better wine.'

I find it hard to believe that multinational alcohol companies beholden to their shareholders would be quite so philosophical if, as a nation, we suddenly decided to drink like the parish vicar. If it doesn't matter how much people drink, why does the industry fight any form of intervention that might lead to a reduction in consumption? 'What the industry objects to most strongly is a group of people with fairly strong agendas coming in and saying, "We think we know best for the rest of you." We don't actually lead or control how much people drink. It's up to people, and the industry's there to fill that need. The industry works very hard to try and control it, in the main. Bottle stores clamp down really hard on underage drinkers, we try and persuade parents not to buy alcohol for their children, hotels try and do a good job around violence and bad behaviour, but there's a lot of young adults saying, "I want to have a drink. How can you say that you know me better than I know me?"'

I didn't think he'd invoke the nanny-state defence this early on, but there it is: the alcohol-regulation equivalent to Charlton Heston's 'guns don't kill people, people kill people' argument. It reminds me of a billboard erected recently near Richmond Station, in the shadow of the MCG. It reads, 'Alcohol doesn't cause violence. Blame and punish the individual.' Financed through an odd alliance of the Nightclub Owners Forum and the Australian Sex Party, the billboard is designed to promote the notion of individual responsibility and to stop 'unfounded attacks' on the hospitality industry.

The war against the wowser endures. From this libertarian standpoint, if I want to get absolutely hammered on cheap grog and vomit into my handbag of an evening, I should be allowed to do that, with as little interference from the state as possible. My dining companion argues that alcohol is already regulated more heavily than most products, in terms of how it's produced, how and when it can be bought, and to whom it can be sold. He says that it's 'punitively taxed', and that there are tight restrictions on how it can be advertised.

I have to pull him up on this one. I've written many stories about the industry's ineffectual, self-regulated advertising code. The code stipulates that alcohol adverts can't link drinking with sexual success. It's hard to reconcile that with Jim Beam's 'The Neighbours' campaign, which showed topless Swedish sunbathers being stalked by peeping toms. The bourbon-maker's adverts, shown as short clips on television and a longer, more explicit version online, featured two blondes in G-strings applying sunscreen, bouncing on a trampoline, and stripping naked as they're watched through a hedge by 'Stevo next door' and his mates. The message wasn't subtle: drinking bourbon makes the act of sexual stalking not only acceptable, but also much more enjoyable. If I didn't know better, I would have sworn it was 1978 and I was watching a Benny Hill skit. Jim Beam pulled the ads after health commentators branded it one of the most offensive promotions in the industry's history. What was worse, they argued, was that these ads — in which a naked woman states, 'We say, "Aussie, Aussie, Aussie, take off your cozzie"' — were deemed appropriate through a pre-vetting process under the industry's self-governed Alcohol Beverages Advertising Code. Public-health campaigners said the advert only served to prove what they had been saying for years: the alcohol industry could not be trusted to regulate itself. It came after an advert for James Boag's depicted a woman holding a beer while sitting on the stairs with her legs spread, wearing only a coat and her underwear. This, too, passed the code's pre-vetting stage. As one health contact said to me at the time, 'When you see ads like that, you have to think that these guys are taking the piss. Self-regulation is a joke.'

My guest concedes that the Jim Beam campaign showed an 'embarrassing lack of judgement', but says no system is perfect, and the pre-vetting process was tightened in subsequent years.

When I ask if the industry uses advertising to entice children, this alcohol executive can't hide his frustration. 'Can you show me an ad that advertises to children? Are you talking about the advertisements in *Dolly* and *Girlfriend*? No, you can't be, because those magazines don't carry alcohol advertising. But if you ask most parents, they'd tell you that the industry does advertise in those magazines.' He says his industry is increasingly having to defend its advertising against 'the vibe': the low expectations of the industry's ethics, and the concerns of desperately worried parents, regardless of whether alcohol companies are behaving improperly. 'I wish people who say alcohol advertising is causing kids to drink would actually put up an ad and say, "This appeals to children." We could debate that, but as it stands, it's just this easy slur to throw out.'

Although he can't be held responsible for the behaviour of his overseas peers, it's hard to believe that the United Kingdom's Lambrini, with its 'girls just wanna have fun' strapline, advertising a range of sparkling 'wine-style' drinks in flavours such as cherry, peach, and apple and blackcurrant, aimed these products at a mature market. Internal industry documents obtained by the 2009 House of Commons inquiry into alcohol advertising showed that the biggest market for Halewood International's Lambrini, and its fruit-cocktail drink Caribbean Twist, was consumers aged 15 to 24. The company's own focus groups clearly show that the product is regarded by the public as a 'kids' drink', yet a creative brief for Lambrini's 2005 campaign describes its target audience as 18 to 24. The brief states the product is a 'light, easy to drink, affordable (wanna be wine) that gets their night out or in off to a good start. They'll drink bucket loads of the stuff and still manage to last the duration.' The same brief adds: 'Drinking starts early! Early afternoon at the weekend or straight after work Monday to Friday meeting your girly mates and getting on it is the only way forward.' Two years later, a television advert for Lambrini that featured energetic dance routines was described internally as a 'cross between Myspace and *High School the* [sic] *Musical.*'

Given the globalised nature of the alcohol industry, is it beyond the realms of possibility that similar conversations are taking place in advertising agencies for Australian brands? The public-health lobby certainly believes it's happening, although sometimes their paranoia seems unwarranted. There have been times over the last few years of reporting on alcohol where I've seen certain sections of the public-health field become so convinced that the industry deliberately sets out to target children, they're jumping at shadows. When Jim Beam and Bundaberg brought out gift packs of bourbon- and rum-flavoured fudge in 2010 and were accused of trying to lure children into drinking, despite the products being completely non-alcoholic, I had to ask myself if perhaps the jihad on binge drinking had become a bit hysterical.

'They think we set out to recruit the next generation of drinkers, but nothing could be further from the truth because we don't have the financial resources to do it, even if we thought it was a good idea. The reasons people drink and how much they drink are so much beyond the industry's control or influence,' my lunch guest says. 'It's just a laughable idea. I've never seen a report that says, "And how is our long-term drinking-addiction project going?" I just don't think it's happening at all.'

Maybe he's right. Perhaps the public-health boffins and academics are paranoid. They won't be happy until prohibition is introduced, and the multinational merchants of death are in court for child endangerment. Sandra Jones, from the University of Wollongong, one of Australia's leading researchers on teenage binge drinking and a formidable thorn in the industry's side, says that she has every reason to be suspicious. At conferences, she presents her findings on what drives young people to drink, and how marketing affects their choice. Sometimes, there will be alcohol industry representatives in the audience. At one conference in New Zealand, three men wearing suits and carrying briefcases walked in, sat down, and began taking notes during her presentation. They left without talking to her. 'They won't say a word to me while they're there, but the next day they'll put out a press release attacking me and rubbishing my research. They don't want to engage in debate — they just want to shut it down,' she told me at a recent conference. She's been called a liar by members of the industry, but more worrying is her belief that her research is being used as a masterclass by alcohol companies seeking to develop the most successful marketing strategies for products that appeal to young people.

We're past the entrees and on to the mains by the time I get round to asking the alcohol-industry executive about the incident we both know I'm going to bring up. I'm reminded of what my colleague Steve Butcher said about getting the most out of contacts: 'A drunk man says what a sober man thinks.' He's on his second glass of wine. Maybe I should order him another.

The incident has been a prickly point between us for some years. I saw it as proof that the alcohol industry deliberately targets young people; he said it was a beat-up. It was the winter of 2007, and public concern over teenage binge drinking was growing. Figures showed that consumption was up, driven by a spike in pre-mixed spirits. With their bright colours and sweet taste, alcopops were clearly designed to appeal to young drinkers, health gurus claimed. Alcohol companies denied it, and said they were predominantly drunk by men over 25 who liked bourbon-, rum-, and whisky-based pre-mixed spirits.

Then I got a scoop they couldn't argue with. In an extraordinarily frank interview, a marketing executive behind a leading vodka brand told me that cheap, sugary drinks packaged in bright colours were the best way to start young people drinking from an early age. Mat Baxter from Naked Communications, the media agency that marketed the vodka-and-citrus drink Absolut Cut, said the market for pre-mixed spirits — apparently known in the industry as the 'binge drinker' category — was booming. Super-strength versions were particularly popular because they 'get young people drunk faster'. He told me: 'It's one of the few drinks where you don't necessarily know you're drinking alcohol, and that's a conscious effort to make those drinks more appealing to young people. The drinks are very much about masking the alcohol taste. When you're young, your palate is tuned for sugary drinks.' He went on to say that drinks with higher alcohol content dominated the pre-mixed spirits market because they appealed to budget-conscious youngsters, who could buy three 7 per cent drinks and get just as drunk as they would if they bought five drinks at 5.5 per cent. It was the first time anyone in the industry had admitted that young people were deliberately being targeted, and health experts were apoplectic. They said that this whistleblower had exposed the grubby truth about an industry intent on encouraging alcohol abuse from an early age. Nobody from the spirits company or the industry body that represented them returned my calls.

My lunch guest dismisses the incident. He says that Baxter wasn't an industry insider; he was an external marketing flack whose comments were his own and not informed by fact. He doubts that Baxter had ever attended a product design meeting or read any consumer feedback, and believes that Baxter's interview with me was part of a crude publicity stunt. Baxter stopped taking my calls after the furore, so I guess we'll never know what he was thinking. But we do know this: whatever the industry's intention, kids are fond of alcopops. A month after the incident, I obtained previously unreleased figures that showed 14- to 19-year-olds at high risk of injury or death through binge drinking preferred pre-mixed alcopops over other drinks. Almost 78 per cent of girls and 74 per cent of boys at risk of short-term harm — of being injured or assaulted, blacking out, overdosing, or dying by drinking six to 11 drinks in one sitting — said that they preferred the pre-mixed spirits over other drinks. Beer was almost as popular with boys, but for girls alcopops were favoured over beer and wine.

It was hardly a surprise. While I know some people my age who drink bourbon and Coke in cans, I can't think of many over the age of 25 who drinks those sickly-sweet fruity drinks.

My lunch guest defends alcopops, saying it's a term that covers both the fruit-flavoured drinks and the cola drinks, and that many adults like the taste and convenience of pre-mixed drinks. As adults, they're entitled to choose these products — and what's the difference between a bottle of spirits, and mixers from the supermarket? Besides, how is the industry to stop teenagers from drinking, when the biggest suppliers of alcohol to underage drinkers are parents?

There were no alcopops to sweeten the revolting taste of alcohol when I started drinking — which probably explains why my friends and I resorted to drinking straight martini (the sweetest drink we could find) as if it were lemonade. Perhaps that suggests kids who want to get drunk will find a way, whatever's on the market. Still, I wonder if making booze more appealing and accessible to young people has encouraged some to drink at an earlier age than they might have if their only option was to put sugar in their beer and swig it through a straw with two fingers pinched over their nose.

As my lunch with a man who is part of the same industry I worked in for more than a decade draws to a close, I'm left pondering our collective role in the social fallout from the nation's alcohol problem. Intentionally or not, we have both fostered it, him through marketing booze to consumers, and me through serving punters in bars. And as clamour grows over how to tackle an epidemic of binge drinking, the industry, willingly or otherwise, is changing. In Melbourne, a freeze on late-night licences means that no new bars, pubs, or nightclubs opening after 1.00 a.m. will be allowed in the city's popular drinking areas until at least the middle of 2013. Across Victoria, all-night bottle shops have had their hours slashed, and the director of liquor licensing now has powers to ban bars from offering cheap-drink promotions that encourage reckless drinking. Fifteen such promotions have been banned since 2009. Nationally, taxes have been raised on alcopops, and some alcohol companies have stopped producing super-strength brands in response to concerns over binge drinking.

The impact of these changes remains to be seen. There's some evidence to suggest that all the alcopops tax achieved was to shift young drinkers to buying bottles of spirits that they mix themselves, arguably a more risky practice than consuming pre-mixed drinks. As Robin Room told me, when it comes to policies that will exact real change in our drinking culture, what works isn't popular and what's popular doesn't work. It might protect problem drinkers to set a minimum price for alcohol, or to introduce a volumetric tax (where the most potent drinks cost more), but the average punter's not going to be impressed when the price of their beer or wine is suddenly hiked up. And when you consider the $5.8 billion in alcohol taxes pouring into the government's coffers each year, you also have to wonder if perhaps some of our leaders think that encouraging people to drink less is not necessarily in the national interest. In a nation bathed in booze, it will be a brave government that tries to pull the plug.

September

IT'S BEEN MORE than two months since I visited Jon Currie and he shook up my world with the words 'pre-malignant addiction'. If damage has been done, I want to know. But the public-health system moves slowly — I'm still waiting for an appointment.

I can hardly complain; I'm not a real patient. Still, the longer I have to wait, the more time there is to dwell on the possible outcome. What if the results of these tests reveal that I have more in common with Jon's patients than I can accept? And why does the thought of drinking again scare me just as much as the thought of not drinking again?

Moderate drinking is probably not an option if I have a damaged brain. And I'm not even sure I want to drink moderately: there are times when I really miss being drunk. I'm a little bored of always being in control; I want to surrender to the night and be taken on a journey. I want to see the 'wonderful, curious things' that Oscar Wilde spoke of so fondly. I don't miss the messy, crying-into-warm-flat-beer-at-5.00-a.m. kinda drunk, but I do hanker for that liquid gold feeling when you're a few drinks in, your inhibitions slowly dissolve, and you share a common buzz with your friends.

Most days, I don't feel cheated because the upside to sobriety is a surprisingly lush plain. I have newfound confidence and a fitter body and mind, and in place of procrastination I have acquired the ability to get shit done. But lately, approaching the pointy end of my year-long sojourn from the sauce, there are times when I really feel the strain. It's hard not to drink for this long, when practically everyone you know drinks regularly. It's hard to stay on track, when alcohol seems to ambush you on every street corner. Sometimes I'm just plain bored. There's something quite liberating about allowing yourself a night where you say, 'Fuck it; I'm going to get smashed.' It's a tension-buster and a reward.

Yesterday, at the end of a long week, there were staff drinks at work and I found myself with my nose buried in a colleague's empty beer bottle, inhaling the enticing smell of Crown Lager. You know you're really missing booze when even the sniff of a Crownie has you salivating. My sense of smell is more keenly attuned to the aroma of alcohol than ever before. On the way home from work, I can sniff out a passenger's lunchtime shiraz from the other end of the tram. When I asked my picture editor recently if she'd had a liquid lunch, she was taken aback. She hadn't touched a drop. I'd picked up the faint smell of alcohol from a home-baked rum ball she'd eaten earlier in the day. My friends have grown accustomed to me sniffing their wine and beer before they have a sip. I close my eyes and inhale the rich fumes, as if trying to recapture the scent of a lover who has slipped away from me.

At night, I often dream of booze. The same recurring theme: I have fallen off the wagon. Sometimes it's in spectacular fashion — vomiting on a bathroom floor or waking up dizzy with shagger's hair and a strange man in my bed. In each dream I am bereft. When I wake, the sense of relief that I have not broken my booze ban is palpable, and this powers me forward. I like to think that these dreams are signposts, as I feel my way in the dark through a foreign land. They point to how gross that Crownie would taste on my breath the morning after a massive night and a few hours' sleep. They point to the fleeting satisfaction of the quick fix.

But this obsession with booze, or the lack of it, makes me fearful. I wonder if these signposts point not only to my past, but also to my future. When I do finally relinquish control, how will I manage freedom? If my hedonistic streak has a more clinical explanation, that freedom might turn into a straitjacket, locking me into an old life I've spent more than eight months trying to change.

I've told close friends about my conversation with Jon Currie. Some find the idea that I might have a dependency on alcohol preposterous. I'm a high-functioning professional woman; I'm not what an addict looks like. Alcoholics drink whisky in brown paper bags; they stumble over and slur their words, lost in a hazy dreamscape. They live in squalor, or they might live well but hide their disease, drinking vodka in the bathroom before the kids get up. But perhaps those perceptions are false — a Hollywood version of what it means to be hooked. Addiction isn't always so clear-cut.

Today, I meet someone who lived a long time in that grey space between sobriety and addiction. Will is a 41-year-old airline engineer from Melbourne. At 3.00 a.m., on a long night shift in April, he'd finished servicing the jets on his list and sat down in a quiet room for a break. He pulled out his iPhone and started to catch up with the day's news. As he scrolled through stories, he found the article about my break from drinking. He told me, 'I was high-fiving the air and saying, "Yes!" out loud. Everything you were writing was me.'

It's been just over two years since Will left rehab. We've spoken on the phone and by email over the last few months, but never met in person. Today, I'm anxious as I come face to face with a man who has been through treatment for an alcohol problem, yet thinks we are living parallel lives. He's a big man, with a gentle demeanour and a permanent smile. His handshake is firm and friendly. We're sitting in the upper atrium of the *Age* building, away from the bustle of the cafe downstairs. I joke that I'm meeting more heavy drinkers sober than I ever did when I was pissed. He laughs and says that, like me, he never thought he'd find himself at the point he's reached, as a non-drinker after so many years of partying. 'My journey to the "High Sobriety" club was a mammoth one,' he says, and I bristle at the name, thinking I've inadvertently formed a Christian prayer group.

His story starts out similarly to mine, although he'd turned 17 before he had his first drink. He saw it as a sign that he was maturing, becoming a man. By the time he reached his twenties, his drinking had become 'professional'. At 23, after stacking on a lot of weight, he decided to give up the grog and go on a fitness kick. He enjoyed his trimmer, sober self. Then, when he earned his engineer's licence, he had what he describes as a 'fuck-it moment', getting on the piss to celebrate. He'd lasted nine months without booze — almost exactly where I am now. As the weeks and months progressed, his old drinking habits crept in. Four beers twice a week became five beers three times a week, then six, seven, eight beers, until he was drinking a dozen beers a day. But that was okay because 'I was the bumbling, happy, fun, silly drunk. Everyone loved me. Life was fun.'

His thirties sneaked up, and it wasn't long before he found himself knocking back 18 cans of VB every day. Some days he might only drink ten beers, but they'd be followed by a bottle of gin. He never drank at work, but he knows there were days when he was impaired, and he frequently drove while over the limit. He was never pulled over. The thought of what could have been still haunts him.

When he came home from work, he'd down a can before he'd even taken his uniform pants off. He drank in front of the television. He drank down the pub with mates. Often he drank alone. His partner of 15 years asked him to cut down, and he would — for a day or two. It didn't last. Only later, during counselling in treatment, did he learn that she'd packed her bags on more than one occasion. Having convinced himself that he didn't have a problem, he was oblivious. But the 'dead soldiers' on bin night were hard to ignore. 'When you go to the pub, you don't see it because you're just drinking a glass. The glass goes, it's refilled, and you continue on again. There's no evidence left behind, which is probably the danger of the pub.'

At his local, he met similar souls. 'When you have a group of heavy drinkers at the pub, they have a bond, a kinship, and they're able to talk about their problems without talking about them directly. That's a very male thing, I guess. Those people were my family. You'd sit at the bar and have a chat about life, about philosophy.'

Will's pub family reminds me of some of the regulars at The Rose. The sense of community has its benefits: mateship and social cohesion, an antidote to loneliness. But it can also harbour denial. When your problem is mirrored back at you in the faces of your friends, it's no longer a problem; it's normal. 'I had some friends who liked to drink with me because they saw me as worse than them. They had their own problems, clearly, but I think it gave them self-confidence because they could look at my drinking and think they weren't that bad. But then, I could always find someone who was worse than me, someone who was another level of severe.'

As the year of his 40th birthday approached, Will's health started deteriorating rapidly. Burdened by huge weight gain and the beginnings of a nervous breakdown, he finally sought help. He told his GP that he felt like he was dying. 'Physically, my body was shutting down. I had trouble breathing, my mind was a mess, I wasn't thinking straight, I wasn't performing like I used to. It was severe. He took a blood test. My liver was looking bad, my blood pressure was really up — everything pointed towards me being in real trouble. I was here at this low point, knowing it was a fork in the road. Turn left and die, turn right and live.'

Even then, he still didn't identify as an addict. He thought that he'd just stop drinking, have some counselling, and get on with things. He was a tough, no-nonsense Aussie bloke who was going to beat this on his own terms. After regular visits with a psychologist, Will reluctantly agreed to enter a private rehab facility. He had to share a room, a big ask for a fiercely private person. Inside this facility, where drug- and alcohol-addled ghosts drifted in the corridors, he was convinced that he was different.

The first few days were boring. 'I didn't really partake in any of the programs; I didn't really seem like I fitted into it. I don't know if it was day three or day four, but I had breakfast, and afterwards I just sat on a couch and played games and read magazines because there's not much to do. Then, I just started to feel like shit. It was nothing like I've ever felt before. It was just getting worse and worse. I was shaky, itchy inside — you feel curly. But it was frightening; it scared the shit out of me. I said to the nurse, "I think I'm not well. There's something wrong with me." I thought I had a cold or something. And they said, "It's starting." I was a mess. I was like that for weeks. My mate who dropped me off came round to see me and I was just a shaking ball.'

The physical withdrawal took Will by surprise. He knew drinking had compromised his body to the point that it was failing him, but he had no idea of the extent of his problem. 'I didn't believe I was bad enough that I needed to go to rehab. You think of rehab and you think of movie stars taking cocaine, and I thought, no, I'm not like that. You don't believe it because it's just alcohol.'

He left rehab after three weeks, but it would take six months for the shakes to stop completely. He knew that he could never drink again. Yet staying on track meant dismantling his old life. It was a 'brutal cut' to ditch his old drinking buddies, and it was painful to avoid the pub, particularly on a warm summer's day, when his mind would taunt him with the sight, taste, and smell of cold beer. Now, he rarely goes to parties. If he does, he creates a 'plan of attack' to protect himself from temptation. It always involves leaving early. 'Drinking puts you in a psychological or behavioural mode, and if you don't have synergy with that mode then you're not part of the party. You've just got to learn to find other ways in life.'

This makes me sad. Is it really the case that you can be the life and soul of the party or you can be a non-drinker, but you can't be both? As much as I try to convince myself that wild times and sobriety are not mutually exclusive, I relate to Will's experience. There's no escaping the imbalance in synergies when you're sober at a party and everyone else is on the piss. Sometimes it's less pronounced than others, and you can dance like a whirling dervish, whooping it up as if you've just knocked back six tequila shots, but other times you have that feeling your immersion is incomplete. After the first few months of this sobriety adventure, I was convinced that I didn't need alcohol to be outrageous and uninhibited. But the longer I abstain, the harder it is to believe that fully. Sometimes, without a drink in my hand, I feel like a pale imitation of that riotous party girl I once was. I miss the freedom of being drunk; I'm nostalgic for the unique sense of merriment you share with fellow drinkers. It's fun and unpredictable in a way that sobriety can't easily replicate. Often, my nights out feel tame in comparison to days of old. There are times when I wonder if my sober self has become imbued with a hint of beige.

For Will, giving up grog meant that he had to redefine his identity. He's no longer the bumbling, fun guy, always ready to crack open a beer with his mates. His new personality is still in its infancy, but just as he once identified as the drunk party animal, now sobriety defines him. 'I had a very distinguished person say to me at work that I was a disgrace for not drinking, and I was so proud of that. As shocking as it was, and the mixed emotions it brought up, jeez, it was a trophy. I'm a totally new person. I would take that over my old identity any day of the week. I'm looking forward to what I can achieve in life.'

But as I listen to him tell me about the things that fill his new life — pottering around the house doing odd jobs, catching up with friends for coffee, and leaving parties early to treat himself to a slice of cake on the way home — it sounds so conservative and controlled. He's moved from that grey space between addiction and sobriety, into a world that is a different shade of grey. But for him, there is no other way. 'I can't drink moderately. That frightens me. If I had one sip of one beer it won't be that Saturday I'll be back into the 18 cans again, but I can see myself slipping into oblivion. It gives you the confidence that you can have one and that's fine. And then next month, something special comes along and you end up having two. And you get confident about that, and this may go on for a year or so, and after five years you're back to 18 cans a day again. That's a reality for me, and there's a very thick, deep line in the sand and I will not cross it. I will not have one. I avoid it. That's the strategy I live with. I will have to do this for the rest of my life, and it's a battle that I may lose one day. But I'm fairly determined. I want to live; I don't want to die a horrible, painful death.'

Still, as he speaks of the fragility of his own mortality, he equivocates when asked if he thinks he's an alcoholic. He stresses that his doctor classified him as a heavy drinker, not an alcoholic. In rehab, he didn't believe the term was an apt description. And now? 'In some capacity, by some classification, to some degree, I'm an alcoholic. Maybe not the classic category-five alcoholic, but in some manner I am.'

I'm astonished that someone who was drinking 18 cans of beer every day, and has been through withdrawal that left his body wracked by tremors, is talking about degrees of addiction. When I stopped drinking, I had no unpleasant symptoms. I felt better immediately. Yet, as we wind the interview up and the conversation shifts to my abstinence, it's clear that he sees me as a kindred soul. He asks if I'll go back to drinking when my year is up. I don't know how to answer. As I umm and aah, his eyes fix on mine and, for the first time in more than an hour, he's not smiling. His expression is urgent. 'You have to ask yourself, who do you want the new Jill Stark to be? Is this Jill Stark happier than the old one? Do you like yourself more now or before?' It's an avenue I'm not comfortable exploring with a relative stranger, but then I look at the notepad resting on my knees and see the most intimate details of his private life. I tell him that I'm definitely happier now. I've gained a lot from not drinking, but I'm hoping I can find a middle ground. Ideally, I'd like to drink moderately, but I worry that my track record suggests I'm no good at this. I don't tell him that I've been fantasising about getting drunk.

It's hard to imagine a life without the occasional Saturday-night blowout, I say. It's how I've lived for 20 years. It's how my friends live. He tells me that I'll have to learn to be brutal with my friends. 'It will take two years to change the social structure around Jill Stark,' he says. 'It's the rock climber–ambulance driver scenario. If you hang around with rock climbers, they're going to tell you how sensational it is — the exhilaration, the fun; they're going to tell you it's such a thrill and you'll really love it. If you hang around with ambulance drivers, they're going to tell you about the broken bones they see, the horrible injuries, the deaths.'

I don't begrudge him the sermon. This man hit rock-bottom only to find there were seven layers of hell hidden in the basement. Like many who embark on that journey, he can't bear the thought of anyone else suffering the same fate. Just as he took his drinking to the extreme, his passion for sobriety has an intensity that borders on evangelism. He doesn't mean to, but the pressure he places on me when he says, 'Jill, I really hope you don't drink again,' is heavy. I don't know if he's pleading for me or for himself. He's co-opted my story as his own. I don't want the responsibility of my sobriety somehow being tied to his.

He tells me that he wants to be an ambassador for people battling alcohol problems. 'My message that I've got from all of this is that there needs to be more of a campaign of watching your mates.

Watch your family, watch your friends, because they're people like me, who do slip into oblivion. People like us, who used to go out and get hammered on a Friday night — it evolves into a bigger problem for us.'

At the time, when he says 'people like us', I think he's referring to others like him, who have sought treatment for a drinking problem. Listening back to my tape later, I'm not so sure. In his eyes, we are both lifelong members of the 'High Sobriety' club. Or at least we should be. But despite the respect and admiration I have for this man, who has overcome such challenges and now wants to share that wisdom, I don't think we're the same. I've never felt the need to drink every day. I can't conceive of a future in which my daily routine would include knocking back half a bottle of gin or the best part of a slab of beer. But I don't suppose Will ever imagined himself that way, either. He's a professional, high-functioning man with a stable home life, whose binge drinking got away from him. He's only seven years older than me. Who knows where I would have been seven years from now if I hadn't taken this step back?

I'VE BEEN INVITED to judge a short-story competition run by Odyssey House, one of Australia's largest drug and alcohol treatment centres. When the entries arrive in the mail, I'm impressed by the standard of writing. The work is supposed to be fictional, but many of the stories are so searing and visceral, they could only have come from lived experience.

Entrants must include reference to alcohol or drugs in the piece, and write to the theme 'how did I get here?' One writes about a teenager's reluctant visit to her father. There are marijuana plants growing on his balcony, and he smokes a bong in front of her with a stoned friend. Another tells the story of a woman whose gambling debts spiral out of control. The narrator mocks the positive-thinking, 'life is for living' messages she sees on television and in magazines.

'Life is where you end up and you just get through all the shit the best you can. Right now, I'm up to my neck in it, and the shovel I've got has a very short handle.' One story, told from the perspective of a boy whose mother died of a drug overdose, conveys his confusion and terror as he's placed in the care of the state when his father, also an addict, is sentenced to 12 years in jail for armed robbery.

But the standout winner moves all three judges to tears. It's the story of an out-of-control 15-year-old girl. She hides vodka in her school locker and turns up to class stoned. There has been no love in her life. When Maryann, a motherly addiction counsellor, tries to reach out to her, she runs away, seeking solace in the bed of a nameless stranger: 'My heart had no room for anyone — not even me.' But slowly she learns to trust Maryann, and reveals the secret of her sexual abuse. This story, hauntingly real and yet remarkable in its restraint, is made all the more poignant when we learn that it's a eulogy to Maryann, who passed away not long after coming into the girl's life. Yet, despite the grief, she finds a way out of her hopelessness and goes on to have a family of her own, ending the story with a question: 'How did I get so lucky?'

In a meeting at Odyssey House Victoria's Richmond head-quarters with the other judges — author and child-protection campaigner Barbara Biggs, and Odyssey's chief executive Stefan Gruenert — we are unanimous in our decision. It leaves me thinking of this young woman's struggle, and I realise something. My 'fuck it, I just want to get smashed' moments are usually about boredom and pleasure-seeking. When I get drunk, it's a choice. For so many others, it's about obliteration — a way to block out the pain. Yet, despite the tragic circumstances that cause already vulnerable people to seek solace in a bottle or through a needle, as a community we still treat addiction as if it's a character failing. How often do we turn our heads as we judge the unpleasant-smelling man staggering through the train carriage? It's funny how we view public drunkenness as socially unpalatable if it's an old man drinking Scotch from a brown paper bag, but it's a bit of fun if it's a group of young women causing a commotion on a hen's night. It makes me wish, once again, that I'd shown more compassion to my granddad. I was young, but I still judged him.

After we make our decision, I stay behind to chat to Stefan. The stories we've read are real life for many of the people he sees in treatment at Odyssey House. He hopes that this inaugural short-story competition will encourage others to share their experiences of drug and alcohol addiction. The stigma of substance abuse is fairly entrenched, he says, but it's slowly changing. Those who have long toiled in this unglamorous sector of health prevention and rehabilitation are starting to see a shift, both here and overseas — people struggling with addiction are choosing to waive anonymity and to publicly celebrate their road to recovery. They and others are giving addiction a visible presence, through walks organised by groups such as the United Kingdom's Recovery Academy, and Faces and Voices of Recovery in the United States. Melbourne's first recovery walk is scheduled for 2012. Central to the movement's philosophy is that everyone's road out of addiction will be different and, to borrow a cliché, recovery is not a destination but a journey.

'Previously, recovery had a whole lot of baggage around it. It was just the Alcoholics Anonymous 12-step program, and you had to say, "I'm an alcoholic or a drug addict and I will be for life, and I'm going to completely give up." It worked for a lot of people, but it wasn't very inclusive,' Stefan says. 'Recovery's now much broader, less concerned about the definition and more a movement for people to celebrate wellbeing and change, and for inspiring others to think about their quality of life. Whether you're still using or not, you can be in recovery — even if you're working towards it.'

By lifting the veil on addiction, in the same way that mental illness is slowly being demystified, the hope is that more people will seek help, and that the public will come to view substance dependency as they do any other medical condition. 'You don't have cancer and [feel as if you have to] be anonymous, and that's part of the shift,' Stefan says. 'All of the self-help fellowship movements have been very underground and hidden because of the shame and stigma. It just feels like the timing's right for people who have their own personal journeys of addiction to suddenly be okay to start sharing their stories and not lose their job or fear that that's going to hurt them. We're at the start of some upswing here, where you'll see more of the people like Ben Cousins — not just the high-profile people but at all levels of society — sharing their story in workplaces and at barbecues, saying, "Actually, I had issues years back and I'm better now."'

When Cousins, one of the AFL's biggest stars and arguably one of the greatest to ever play the game, had his very public fall from grace, there were many lining up to condemn him. He had fled a booze bus, spent time in a Los Angeles rehab clinic, and been arrested for drug possession, which led to a 12-month playing ban for bringing the game into disrepute. He was a supremely talented, wealthy young man with Hollywood good looks, who seemed to be throwing it all away for the sake of a party. Yet, following a screening of a documentary outlining Cousins' battles with substance abuse, Channel Seven invited Australian Drug Foundation chief executive John Rogerson to explain the complexities of addiction to the audience at home. For Rogerson, and for many others in the field, it was a sign that addiction was starting to be taken seriously by mainstream media, and to be viewed as a health problem rather than a lifestyle choice.

But sometimes the spotlight can be a curse. As more people seek help, treatment services are buckling under the weight of demand. Between 2000 and 2010, there was a 29 per cent increase in the number of publicly funded treatments for drug and alcohol problems in Australia, with booze being the principal drug of addiction in nearly half (48 per cent) of all cases, up from 37 per cent of cases in 2000. These figures don't include those who drink heavily while using another drug. In Victoria, the Salvation Army estimates that the drug and alcohol treatment sector is already under-funded by at least 50 per cent. Nationally, the situation's no better. Those in the sector complain that politicians are quick to allay middle-class paranoia about violent smackheads and the rise of illegal drugs, however spurious the evidence, but are loath to tackle a legal substance that wreaks widespread havoc — perhaps because it's a drug that most voters enjoy on a regular basis.

A senior drug and alcohol–sector professional told me that they were once forced to sit next to a politician at a press conference, nodding in stony-faced agreement as the pollie announced a multi-million-dollar crackdown on methamphetamine. The money came after a series of hysterical and largely unfounded stories in sections of the media that claimed there had been a massive spike in the use of the drug, often known as 'ice', 'meth', or 'crystal meth'. There was a heightened level of concern about this nasty substance, which can cause users to be aggressive and delusional. Yet there was no evidence of an ice epidemic on the streets of Melbourne. Still, when the government comes knocking, you don't turn them away. They smiled for the cameras and accepted the funds. Then, much of the money was spent where it was needed most — in alcohol-treatment services.

In 2008, Labor announced that $53 million was to be committed to a national binge-drinking strategy, to be rolled out over four years from 2009. But much of the money has gone to anti-drinking campaigns and early intervention for young people; very little has been spent on the treatment sector. Like other rehab facilities across Australia, Odyssey House has experienced a massive increase in the number of people presenting with alcohol problems in the last decade. At any given time, there can be 100 or more people waiting for a place in Odyssey's residential rehabilitation facilities. Stefan says that only about 10 per cent of people with a drinking problem will seek help, compared to up to 80 per cent of those with an illicit drug habit. When people reach that fork in the road, just as Will did — where left means oblivion and right means survival — they can easily be hurried down the wrong path if there's a long wait for treatment. Will was fortunate that he could afford a private facility, but even then he waited several weeks before a place in residential rehab came up.

In the public system, the situation is dire. Demand grows exponentially every year. I'm reminded of a man who left a comment online, underneath my binge-drinking story, in April. He'd been fighting alcoholism for 26 years. 'I wish I could give up for a few days let alone a few months or a lifetime … my liver is getting more fragile and I can tell brain damage is setting in. I'm not stupid … [I] have two degrees, teaching at university and about to start a PhD.' He lamented the lack of publicly funded treatment options for those with alcohol addiction, predicting that he'd have to get much more seriously ill before being offered support. 'Of course, if I get taken out of my house in a body bag I'll be sadly beyond help.'

As more people find the confidence to speak up about their battles with alcohol, Stefan fears that a system already at breaking point will be swamped. 'We're getting a lot of people in their mid to late thirties, but we're also getting people right into their sixties, and I think that's going to be another emerging issue among older Australians. We've got a growing cohort of people going to be entering aged care, and a lot of them have had drinking patterns all their life that have been pretty unhealthy. How are we going to manage those people?'

At the other end of the spectrum is a young generation of drinkers who have grown up in a culture that embraces excess and teaches them to mark every life event with alcohol. For most teens, binge drinking won't lead to dependency. But for some, it's the gateway to addiction. The number of young people being treated for alcohol-related brain damage grew five-fold in a decade. Arbias, one of Australia's only treatment services for brain injuries caused by drinking, saw the number of patients aged 16 to 25 jump from 120 in 1997 to 600 in 2007.

A few years ago, I spent the day with the Youth Substance Abuse Service, Victoria's biggest treatment and support service for 12- to 25-year-olds. I visited its residential rehabilitation centre and drop-in day program in Fitzroy, an area traditionally associated with high rates of drug and alcohol problems. About 30 young people, mostly under the age of 21, visited it daily. I like to think I'm a fairly worldly-wise person, but I was shocked by what I found. There were kids there who had suffered unimaginable neglect and abuse. Some of them sold themselves on the street to feed their habit; many were homeless. When the centre opened its doors in the late 1990s, heroin was the main problem, but now, overwhelmingly, it's alcohol. In a decade, the number of young people being treated for alcohol dependency has doubled. Some are so hooked they're drinking a slab of beer or two bottles of spirits a day.

After I leave Odyssey House, I go back to the Youth Substance Abuse Service, now known as the Youth Support and Advocacy Service, to see what's changed. I arrive at the Fitzroy residential withdrawal centre — an eight-bed facility for young people detoxing from alcohol and other drugs — and a support worker invites me into the living area, as I wait for chief executive Paul Bird to make his way over from the YSAS office nearby. It's a colourful space that feels like a big share house, with a pool table, couches, beanbags, and a pinboard filled with photographs of young people smiling and pulling faces. A punching bag hangs in the courtyard.

A guy, wearing a baseball cap and baggy jeans, walks past the dining table, where I'm waiting. He scowls at me as we make eye contact. He's gaunt and pale. Despite the tough exterior, he has a child's face — he can't be much older than 16.

When Paul arrives, I'm keen to know what kinds of back-grounds the kids who come here for help have. As it was when I last visited, he says that most of them come from broken homes, have been in trouble with the police, or have experienced homelessness. What's changed is that the service is now seeing more young people who came to Australia as refugees from Africa and Afghanistan, and have lost their way in our drinking culture. Alcohol abuse is so rife in those communities that the centre recently closed its doors to new referrals for a week to look after young Sudanese men exclusively.

'Their parents have come from a stricter culture, where drinking and substance use are not practised regularly, and then they arrive here, to a very open culture, and they're all of a sudden put in an Australian school with Australian friends. Their friends are completely different from their family, so you see family breakdown as well,' Paul tells me. 'They may have greater ties to community groups, but not to their parents and elders, so they kind of go from nought to 60 very fast. You see very heavy substance use in a very short period of time, and that's causing massive issues with anger and violence, not to mention that alcohol and drugs are used as a way to escape from the trauma they've experienced in their homeland.'

It's not surprising that these new Australians, suddenly furnished with freedom and access to cheap booze, would mimic the ways of their adopted country. And it almost certainly doesn't help that many migrants are being housed in already disadvantaged areas, such as Greater Dandenong, in Melbourne's south-east, which has the second-highest youth unemployment rate in Victoria.

But the increase in demand for treatment is not just in underprivileged communities. The YSAS helpline increasingly fields calls from parents in Melbourne's growth corridors. In these outer suburban areas, where there are inadequate or often non-existent public-transport links and few after-school activities for young people, excessive drinking is a burgeoning problem. Paul says: 'People have moved there to get a bigger house. They see the developers' adverts, they see images of people frolicking in fields, and they go there as a lifestyle choice — and suddenly they've got a very big house, mortgaged to the hilt, their commute times have increased, both parents are at work, so the kids come home from school alone. They may end up with another peer group who doesn't go straight home from school, and that's where disengagement comes from. The stress, financially, is so great that families are just breaking up, but they still look prosperous because they've got big houses, they've got the McMansions. There's a kind of facade that there's wealth and wellbeing there, but if you look behind it, nobody sees that.'

Paul says, too, that while boredom, frustration, and the risk-taking nature of teenagers can contribute to them turning to alcohol, it's also behaviour they learn from their parents, many of whom drink to cope with financial and relationship problems. 'In the past, [parents] may have had the social connections to deal with this, but now they're living in the outer suburbs, they have less connection. They're less engaged with their kids, and they're not established in local football or the myriad things that more-established suburbs have. There's more alcohol use, and anger and violence in the family, and learned behaviours that the kids have picked up as a result of their environment.'

Despite the increase in alcohol and drug problems in these communities, services like YSAS are trying to cater for such growing suburbs without extra funding. In six years of health reporting, I've watched the treatment sector buckle under the weight of seemingly never-ending growth in demand. Governments have talked tough on cracking down on alcohol-related violence and teenage binge drinking, yet those at the sharp end of the problem continue to flounder, with limited money to help those most in need. In March

2011, Victoria's auditor-general released a damning report, asserting that the state's drug and alcohol treatment system was chronically under-funded, after successive state Labor governments had failed to act on 31 system reviews over the last decade. As the politicians sat on their hands, waiting times for residential rehab had doubled. The report also revealed a revolving-door system, with 70 per cent of those treated later re-admitted, after suffering a relapse. And not only has funding failed to keep pace with the growth in demand, but it has actually gone backwards in terms of per-capita spending.

When former premier John Brumby released his much-vaunted Alcohol Action Plan for Victoria in 2008, it committed $14 million to awareness campaigns and help for GPs to support people with drinking problems, but gave no new funding to the treatment sector. The Baillieu government has pledged to address the problem, but services such as YSAS and Odyssey House won't see any new cash until the completion of a long public-consultation process — essentially, another system review.

In the meantime, I wonder what will happen to the teenagers who drink themselves into oblivion night after night, and find there's nowhere to go when they have a moment of clarity that gives them the impetus to seek help. How many of those disaffected kids in the outer suburbs will slip from binge drinking to dependency, when proper support might have prevented that trajectory?

It must be unbelievably frustrating for those who see firsthand how vital it is to treat addiction early. Awareness campaigns are simply not enough. But there is hope. They're buoyed by the rise of the recovery movement, and by youth-led organisations such as *Hello Sunday Morning*, which celebrate those who choose not to drink. They hope that, just as the boozy photos and status updates on Facebook create a social-contagion effect, the growing numbers of young people talking about taking a break from drinking or going teetotal will have a ripple effect in peer groups.

There's some evidence that this is already happening. It doesn't make the headlines, but there are a growing number of young people who are staying sober or delaying their first drink. The Australian School Students Alcohol and Drug Survey, which is carried out every three years and is considered the most reliable gauge of substance use in young people, shows that the number of 12- to 17-year-olds who had never had an alcoholic drink grew from 12 per cent in 2002 to 18 per cent in 2008, when the last survey was conducted. The 2010 National Drug Strategy Household Survey recorded that 77 per cent of 12- to 15-year-olds had not had a drink in the previous 12 months — up from 70 per cent in the 2007 survey. Among 16- to 17-year-olds, the proportion who had not drunk in the previous year increased from 24 per cent to 32 per cent over the two surveys.

What may help boost those numbers is the increasing list of celebrities who are proving that you can be sober and cool. British pop star Lily Allen gave up drinking after confessing her wild-child ways were turning her into a 'character in a comic, and that character is always drunk'. In July, Oasis bad boy Liam Gallagher quit booze after '20 years drinking and messing about', and said that it improved his singing voice. And at the tender age of 21, *Harry Potter* star Daniel Radcliffe, hero to millions of children, turned his back on the bottle, saying he'd become too reliant on alcohol. He said he got swept away in the celebrity lifestyle and had been using booze to fit in. More locally, in June, 23-year-old Triple J radio host Alex Dyson became the 1000th person to take on the *Hello Sunday Morning* challenge, with a three-month break from drinking; the publicity from his decision led to an immediate jump in sign-ups.

This is perhaps the most powerful way to change an environment that makes it so difficult for young people to turn down a drink. It's not about telling younger Australians not to drink; it's about promoting the idea that alcohol is something you enjoy, not something you need. As Chris Raine says, 'It's easy to get swept up in a drinking culture. Sometimes we just need a rope to pull us back to dry land.'

The question remains: is that rope strong enough to bear the weight of a generation at risk of being dragged under?

October

BEER, FOOTY, AND a meat pie — it's the Australian way. But as fond as I am of booze combined with saturated fat wrapped in pastry, I haven't always been a fan of AFL. When I first arrived in Melbourne, I was all about the beautiful game. I'd been a diehard football fan since Dad first took me to see Hearts, one of two Edinburgh-based Scottish Premier League teams, when I was ten years old. I couldn't imagine loving any sport more. Football was life. It had flair, finesse, and skill.

All I knew about Aussie Rules football was that it was a tough, take-no-prisoners skirmish that often bore the hallmarks of an all-in pub brawl. It was high-scoring, fast, and physical. But I was unconvinced of its merit. Yet mid-way through the 2001 AFL home-and-away season, when I'd been living in Melbourne for just a few weeks, my then partner, Hugh, took me to footy's church. And there, in the roaring cauldron of the MCG, watching Hawthorn smash Collingwood, I was converted. This was the best game in the world.

It was the beginning of a long and often painful love affair with the Hawthorn Football Club. By the time my relationship with Hugh ended, the brown and gold had seeped under my skin and into my blood. Now, for six months of the year, football is my non-negotiable weekly ritual. It's electrifying, addictive, and at times soul-destroying.

Coming from a country where opposing fans are segregated, and alcohol is banned for fear that the crowd will erupt in violence, I initially found it odd that I could drink at the footy and sit where I liked. But for several years, beers before and at the game with my Hawks friends were part of the tradition — until I stopped drinking. Sometimes, the way Hawthorn play is enough to drive anyone to drink; but this season, sober and lucid, I've realised that my being drunk doesn't make the boys perform any better. When you're losing, that over-priced, mid-strength cooking beer you've been chugging back for four quarters suddenly seems like a massive waste of money. Yet when you're winning ... well, that's a different story.

It's a long-established tradition, both here and where I grew up, to toast sporting success with a drink. Although historically, with the exception of some wins in curling and darts, there's been little to cheer about in Scottish sport, that hasn't stopped us from getting on the piss. One of the most common chants you'll hear from fans when the Scottish national football team plays is, 'Here for the bevvy, we're only here for the bevvy.' So when Hearts beat Rangers to win the Scottish Cup in 1998, ending a 36-year trophy drought, it was a momentous occasion in our house. Dad had been a teenager when he last saw the boys in maroon get their hands on silverware. At the game, I cried tears of joy and relief when I watched my team lift the cup. Then, like most other long-suffering Jambos (Hearts = Jam Tarts = Jambos), I got absolutely hammered. I was pissed for three days. Nobody, not even my moderation-preaching father, questioned it. We'd earned the party.

In 2007, when Geelong won their first AFL premiership in 44 years, it brought back those memories as I watched Loretta and the other friends who had stuck with the Cats through decades of heartache embark on a week-long bender. A year later, I was lucky enough to watch Hawthorn win the flag. Having missed the glory days of the 1970s and 1980s, I hadn't known success as a Hawks fan; since I'd been following them, there were lean years with many woeful performances, and I'd begun to wonder if perhaps I was a jinx. When we won the premiership, the celebrations went on for days. I drank beer by the barrelful and sang the club song until I was hoarse.

Grand-final day in Melbourne is one of my favourite days of the year, regardless of who's playing. For a week leading up to it, the city's buzzing as footy fans wear their colours and prepare to enjoy an epic battle between the season's two best teams. On the day itself, it's okay to crack open a beer at 11.00 a.m., and drunkenness is excused and expected. In ten years of living in Melbourne, I've never experienced the day sober. Even when I was pulling pints at The Rose Hotel, I got on the sauce as soon as I knocked off, catching up quickly with mates who'd been on it all day. Last year there were two chances to get wasted, after the drawn grand final forced a replay. I took full advantage of them.

This year will be different in two ways. The expansion of the league has seen the fixture move from the traditional last Saturday in September to the first Saturday in October. Perhaps more noteworthy to me is the fact that I'll watch the game without a beer in my hand. I've survived the home-and-away season without craving a drink. It's actually been quite liberating not having to queue to buy crap beer in a plastic cup. My abstinence even inspired one of my match-day friends, Sophie, to give up booze for a couple of weeks. But at the preliminary final against Collingwood last week, I doubted whether I would make it through the finals series without a drink. Few had given us a chance against last year's premiers, but halfway through the third quarter, we were on top and dominating. Suddenly, a berth in the grand final was a real possibility. As I chewed my nails and watched through half-open eyes, I was gripped by a vision of Hawthorn captain Luke Hodge standing on the dais with the premiership cup in his hands. How could I not get drunk if we won the flag?

There's something about sporting triumph that just merits alcoholic acknowledgement. Maybe it's because it can be so emotionally draining to achieve it that a boozed-up celebration is the only way to release that tension. Or maybe it's about bonding with friends over a mutual passion. In Australia, it might be due to the weather. Sunshine always makes beer taste better.

But on a structural level, it's much more than that. Alcohol is the lifeblood of every major sport in this country. Whether it's the AFL's 100-year-old partnership with Carlton Draught, the Australian cricket team spruiking VB, or the Formula One Grand Prix partnering with Johnnie Walker, Australian sport is saturated with booze. Of the $119 million spent on advertising by the alcohol industry in 2008, a quarter was linked to sport — Foster's alone spent $20 million in direct deals with the AFL, the NRL, and Cricket Australia. Sporting heroes have become mobile billboards for alcohol companies.

Of course, the industry flatly rejects claims that they use sport to promote excessive drinking, and say that their advertising only affects a consumer's brand choice, not how much they drink. Indeed, I have to say that I'm continually amazed by how convivial the atmosphere is at the football, despite free-flowing beer (albeit mid-strength). It's rare to see people really wasted, and even on grand-final day there are few arrests. There's more violence on the field than in the stands. But I find it hard to believe that alcohol companies have any interest in encouraging moderate drinking. For instance, it's difficult to reconcile Foster's claim to be responsible corporate citizens with their VB promotion in which they gave away a talking doll of former cricket star David Boon (famous, as we've seen, for knocking back 52 beers during a flight from Sydney to London). Programmed to respond to electronic triggers during television coverage of the VB-sponsored one-day series, the doll's favourite catchphrases included, 'When are we going to the pub?' and 'Boony wants some beer.' By the end of the 2006 promotion, more than 200,000 talking dolls had been given away with slabs of VB. Not long after, half-yearly results revealed that Foster's had enjoyed its highest beer sales in a decade.

For many Aussies, these promotions are a laugh. It's harmless fun. And while they might be tempted to buy a slab to collect a Boony doll, it has little bearing on how much they'll actually drink when watching the cricket. Just like the MCG's notorious Bay 13, where rowdy fans get pissed, start Mexican waves, and sledge opposition players, these promotions are all part of the fun of the game. It shows that we're a nation of lovable larrikins who don't take ourselves too seriously.

But public-health experts don't find it funny. They argue that much of the industry's advertising is trying to shore up brand loyalty in a new generation of drinkers. When a giant inflatable pot of Carlton Draught floats across the MCG on grand-final day — as it did in 2008 — casting a colossal shadow on the hallowed turf, kids would be forgiven for thinking that beer is an essential part of their footy experience. The television adverts for the 'official beer of the AFL' are similarly hard to ignore: they're often movie-style, big-budget productions, designed to make you laugh and make such an impact that you'll be talking about them with your friends the next day. Arguably, these ads are just as likely, if not more, to appeal to middle-aged men as kids. But what worries the public-health lobby is growing research that shows early exposure to this type of advertising desensitises children to alcohol and increases the likeliness of underage drinking. The effect appears to be more pronounced when those ads feature their sporting heroes. If Michael Clarke's wearing the VB logo on his cap as he takes a wicket, or the

Wallabies are sharing a rum and Coke with a seven-foot-tall talking polar bear, that's got to be cool. The potential to glamorise booze and encourage underage drinking is the reason that alcohol ads are banned during children's television viewing hours (that is, before 9.00 p.m.). But here's the rub: live sporting events are exempt.

It's a loophole that critics say alcohol companies are exploiting to bombard children with advertising during events they know they'll be watching. This is exactly the type of marketing that my alcohol-industry contact denies is designed to reach a young audience of potential drinkers. A study conducted by the Cancer Council in April 2011 found that 116,000 children under the age of 17 tuned in to watch the Bathurst 1000 V8 Supercars event; in two hours of race coverage, they were exposed to alcohol messages 106 times. They saw ads for Jim Beam, XXXX Gold, Jack Daniel's, Sirromet wines, and bottle-shop chains BWS and The Bottle-O. The images were on the podium, on the track, plastered over the cars, and popping up as on-screen graphics — and all were shown before 8.30 p.m. Leaving aside the appropriateness of partnering hard liquor with an event showcasing fast cars, it does seem that this exemption is a peculiar anomaly for a product that our political leaders claim is turning young people into violent delinquents.

The Australian Medical Association, the Greens, and the Australian Drug Foundation are among groups that want to see alcohol advertising kicked out of sport for good. They want a federal government buy-back of the estimated $300 million that alcohol companies spend on sports sponsorship every year. But each time a ban is raised, the major sporting codes have come out swinging. In a joint submission to a 2007 Senate inquiry into alcohol harm, they claimed that up to 23 per cent of all sport revenue comes from alcohol sponsorship, warning that a ban would decimate community sport and send many grassroots clubs to the wall. Likewise, in 2009, when the Preventative Health Taskforce recommended an end to alcohol companies sponsoring sport, AFL boss Andrew Demetriou said that a ban would 'cripple football'. It's the same argument that cigarette manufacturers used to oppose a ban on tobacco sponsorship in the late 1980s. But the sky is yet to fall in — clubs have found new sponsors.*

In France, where there's been a ban on alcohol advertising since 1991, rugby union's European tournament, the Heineken Cup, was renamed the H Cup to satisfy broadcast regulations. American brewer Anheuser-Busch, which secured world sponsorship rights to the 1998 World Cup in France, tried to have the ban overturned to allow its Budweiser brand to be displayed on pitch-side hoardings. The French government refused to make an exception. The brewer was forced to sell the advertising space, and a new sponsor was found in Japanese electronics company Casio, proving there are alternatives to liquor when it comes to sponsorship.

Here, alcohol experts say we're five or ten years away from such a ban. In a nation obsessed with sport, I'd say it will be much longer. It's hard to imagine what an AFL season would look like without alcohol promotions. There would be no Crownies at the Brownlow, no big-budget beer ads on grand-final day, and 12 out of 18 footy clubs would be looking for a new sponsor.

This season, with drinking removed from my football experience, I've started to notice how insidious these promotions are. Tuning into radio station Triple M, I notice that commentators regularly count a player's match statistics in beer. 'He's not great in the Carlton Draught long-kick department,' James Brayshaw says, in all

---

* As it turns out, in June 2012 sports minister Kate Lundy announced a deal with 12 sporting codes, including soccer, basketball, netball, swimming, and cycling, which saw the organisations share $25 million in government funding in return for agreeing to end all alcohol sponsorship arrangements and to promote responsible drinking. Australia's biggest sporting codes — AFL, cricket, and rugby — did not sign up to the deal. Around the same time, the AFL extended its sponsorship deal with Carlton & United Breweries for another five years. Under fire for wowserism, health minister Tanya Plibersek said that a lot of sport depended on alcohol sponsorship, and that the government had 'no intention of banning alcohol advertising'.

seriousness, to his co-host Garry Lyon on their Saturday-afternoon live commentary. 'No, he's only had three Carlton Draughts for the whole game,' Lyon replies. This word-substitution, part of a sponsorship deal with the brewing giant, might occur a dozen or more times in a two-hour broadcast. When every kick, handball, and goal is measured in beer, what does that say about alcohol's place in competitive sport to a kid who tunes in?

Footy culture is blokey, and I suspect that the idea that sport and drinking are inextricably linked to masculinity is planted in boys' minds from an early age. The more you drink, the more of a man you are. Young men can't fail to notice that some of the most talented AFL players of the modern era — Ben Cousins, Brendan Fevola, and Wayne Carey — have been party boys. But if AFL is seen as a macho sport, where alcohol and testosterone-fuelled bad behaviour are all part of the package, arguably rugby league is even more so. Earlier this year, following a series of alcohol-related incidents involving players from the Sydney Roosters, former league star Wayne Pearce said that the binge-drinking culture was the biggest blight on the game. He warned that the sports stars' behaviour threatened to damage the reputation of the game by sending the wrong message to supporters.

Involvement with local rugby union and league clubs forged a pattern of heavy drinking for 39-year-old Brent, a *Hello Sunday Morning* blogger from Brisbane. When we talk on the phone, he tells me that he had his first beer in the changing rooms at 14, after watching his father play. 'They'd won something, and there were beers going around. Dad gave me a beer, and I thought I was pretty cool. They used to do shotguns, where you stick a key in a can and you have to scull the lot — whoever got the best player did shotguns. When you won trophies, you'd drink beer out of trophies. It was just what everyone did back then.'

By 17, he'd begun playing rugby himself. A big night on the

town was obligatory after the game and after training. Some of the clubs he played with were sponsored by local bars or hotels, and instead of giving the team money for the privilege of having the bar's name on their shirts, the publicans paid them in free drinks. Once a week, the team would descend on the venue to drink their bar tab. Away matches were also swimming with alcohol. 'Every bus trip I've ever been on, for any club I've ever played for, we'll always get booze for the bus trip home — and the longer the bus trip, the more booze you get. You also tend to stop at pubs along the way. I went on a rugby trip in Grade 12 and we were drinking in pubs on the way back. The bus driver and coach were organising our booze when we were 17 years old, so it gets bred into you pretty early.'

He continued to play rugby (league and union) into adulthood, hanging up his boots a couple of years ago. Even in his thirties, the rituals were the same. 'Last time I played was in Mount Isa. We played teams that came from out of town, and after the game we had boat races: you have four or five players in your teams, you nominate your best drinkers, and it's like a relay, so you'll drink a beer and slam it down, the next guy will drink it, and you try and beat the other team. But in Mount Isa, we'd do it with shots of absinthe. You might have a can of beer and a shot of absinthe, and you've got to knock that back, and the next guy goes, and you just try and drink it faster than the other team. The team that finishes first wins.'

Another drinking game popular on trips away was the 100 Club, where players were challenged to drink 100 beers in 100 minutes. Everyone got an empty glass and had to fill up the glass of the teammate next to them. Every minute, someone shouted, 'Drink!' and players had to finish everything in their glasses. If you made it through 100 minutes, you became a member of the 100 Club. On a team trip to Bali ten years ago, the results weren't pretty. 'What happens is, you fill up the guy to the left of you, and you might do that for ten minutes, and then he'll fill up your glass. You can fill it up as full as you like, but you know he's going to have a chance to get you back. And if you can't drink, or if you throw up or you urinate, then you're out. It starts with guys just pouring shots of beer, but towards the end it gets messy and people start filling up glasses, and the last 20 minutes can get a bit full-on. People throw up. They can't handle the volume of beer.'

Alcohol is often used as a way to pump money back into local sports clubs, through sponsorship and selling grog at fundraising events. At his former rugby league club in Brisbane, Brent recalls 'horn and prawn' nights at which, for $100 a ticket, players and supporters would pack into an industrial shed to enjoy seafood, booze, and strippers. It proved to be a successful revenue raiser until the events became rowdy, fights broke out, and community members objected to the overall unseemliness, and they were shut down. While back then, in his twenties, it was 'a bit of a laugh', as the father of a ten-year-old girl, he now views it with regret. Brent thinks that these days local rugby clubs are less reliant on alcohol, and he knows players who don't drink at all during the season — but there's no doubt that he learned to drink by being involved in sport.

So why was alcohol such an integral part of his rugby-playing experience, I wonder. 'The social aspect's quite important: there's a lot of bonding that's done over it. It's all very fraternal,' he says. 'But I suppose it's just all around you. The Australian cricket team drink VB. I've been at the cricket that many times where by lunchtime you're that boozed, you wouldn't have a clue what's going on. You go to the races and you watch the first couple, and for the rest of the day it's a social thing and there's a horse race in the background. It's become such a big part of our culture. Alcohol seems to be sport's vice.'

MY DILEMMA ABOUT whether to drink if Hawthorn won the premiership was short-lived: a last-quarter capitulation against Collingwood saw us lose the preliminary final by three points in the dying minutes. I hadn't been that devastated by a sporting catastrophe since Hearts lost the Scottish Premier League and Cup double in the space of a week, at the end of the 1985–86 season.

After the Hawks went down, I walked back from the MCG in the rain, through a sludge of bullish Collingwood fans, and got home in time to hear our coach, Alastair Clarkson, tell a press conference that the boys just weren't good enough. 'We had them on the ropes and we didn't finish them off,' he said glumly.

Losing was awful. I could only imagine how bad the players felt. After a gruelling six-month season, slugging it out in one of the most physically challenging competitions in the world, they had nothing to show for their efforts but battered bodies and dented pride. It should have been no surprise that some of them went off the rails when it was over.

Whether it's the pressure of the spotlight or the thrill-seeking nature of athletes, who spend their lives pumped with adrenaline, some footballers can't seem to help getting into trouble when they drink. This year started with Brisbane Lions star Brendan Fevola being arrested for drunken bad behaviour; it wasn't his first boozy night of shame. Then in April, Melbourne vice-captain Brent Moloney celebrated his best-on-ground performance in a win over Brisbane by getting so drunk that he was thrown out of a nightclub at 3.00 a.m., just hours before he was due to turn up for training. In 2010, a magistrate had warned Collingwood's Heath Shaw that he was putting his career at risk after he twice got behind the wheel after drinking, despite a court-enforced order that he be completely sober when driving. It followed an incident two years earlier, in which he and teammate Alan Didak were nearly sacked following a boozy night out that saw him crash into several parked cars. In 2009, Essendon rising star Michael Hurley assaulted a taxi driver at 5.30 a.m. in a dispute over a fare, after a night spent drinking at Channel Nine's *The Footy Show* end-of-season revue after-party.

'Mad Monday', the traditional end-of-season piss-up, is also notorious for bad behaviour and excessive drinking. Wary of the publicity and more mindful of their duty of care to the young men in their charge, clubs now manage these events tightly so that players get into less trouble than they once did. But every year, without fail, there will be at least one player who ends up getting arrested for urinating in public; drink-driving; getting into a brawl with a punter; or somehow embarrassing themselves, the club, and the AFL on an alcohol-fuelled night of temporary madness. It's not easy to rein in a group of young men who spend most of the year adhering to a strict training and nutritional regime, and by season's end are raring to cut loose.

A 2009 study in *The Medical Journal of Australia* found that 54 per cent of AFL players drink at levels likely to cause long-term harm during the two weeks following the season's end, and 41 per cent drink that way during vacation times. The same year, Pippa Grange, a psychologist who worked with the AFL Players Association, told me in an interview that nightclubs encouraged this type of drinking, putting on bar tabs for high-profile players to allow them to drink for free to a set limit. 'Sometimes those drink cards can be ridiculously big — as high as $1000. Venues want the footy stars in there because they attract a particular crowd of young people. Because the drinks are free, it's like a smorgasbord — you're just going to keep going back until you're totally over-full or too drunk,' she said.

For the same story, I spoke to former footballers from the 1970s and 1980s, all steeped in a heavy-drinking culture that made getting on the piss an unquestioned part of the game, even during the season. After the final siren, players would share beers in the changing rooms. 'Recovery' sessions the following day were also often boozy affairs, where hardened drinkers were viewed as legends.

For the most part, modern-day players wouldn't dream of binge drinking during the season. Former Western Bulldogs star Scott

West — who was dumped by his club at the end of the 2008 season, and later admitted to going on a month-long drinking binge to cope with the sudden end of his career — told me that he didn't advocate a return to those days, but argued that today's young footy stars need to be given more leeway. 'The demographic of the player now is between 18 and 23, and if you have a look at society, at that age they're all going out and having fun and probably getting into fights, but they're not getting on the front page. The expectation on the players is they're professional 24/7 these days. But there should be room for players to have their time and enjoy themselves.'

In 2009, the AFL and the Players Association launched a formal alcohol policy in a bid to clean up the game's image and create a more responsible attitude to grog. Measures included a crackdown on Mad Monday rituals such as drinking games and pub crawls; the introduction of player education on the harms of binge drinking; and responsible-service-of-alcohol policies at best-and-fairest dinners, presidents' lunches, and corporate functions. But while health experts welcomed the move, saying that it went further than any other sporting code's, they pointed out that it was inconsistent with the league's acceptance of an estimated $5 million in annual sponsorship from alcohol companies — particularly as a 2008 New Zealand study found that athletes whose sports were sponsored by alcohol companies were more likely to binge drink. The study of nearly 1300 sportsmen and women from a range of codes, including rugby, soccer, and cricket, showed that nearly half received free or discounted drinks. Research from Deakin University released earlier in 2011 found similar results, with the authors claiming that athletes may drink more than they would if they were sponsored by non-alcohol brands because they feel indebted to their sponsors, and are exposed to more pro-alcohol messages on uniforms, stadium hoardings, and club merchandise.

At the end of the 2008 season, just a few months before the

AFL's new alcohol policy was due for release, Brendan Fevola — who played for Carlton at the time, which was then sponsored by Carlton Draught — was pictured enjoying end-of-season celebrations at Melbourne's Federation Square. He was drunk, wearing a pink nightie, and had a dildo protruding from his pants. When I pointed out to Pippa Grange that this suggested she had her work cut out for her trying to change footy's boozy culture, she reminded me that Fevola was only one of 850 AFL players, the majority of whom are perfectly well behaved.

As the 2011 grand final between Geelong and Collingwood approaches — a contest I'd be happy for both teams to lose — I wonder how many players will get into trouble at this year's after-parties.

When game day arrives, I'm buzzing, ready to party, and soaking up the atmosphere as the television coverage kicks off with the traditional North Melbourne grand-final breakfast. I'm actually quite looking forward to not drinking, given that some of the worst hangovers I've had have followed these matches.

Unfortunately, my day turns out to be a disappointment. Not because I can't drink, but because I have to work. At midday, I've just stepped out of my apartment with my four-pack of ginger beer, on the way to what promises to be a cracking party with a giant projector screen, when my editor calls to tell me the news. Ironically, I will be kept from the festivities by my own football club's president. There's a story about Hawthorn president and former Victorian premier Jeff Kennett, and his role with the national depression agency beyondblue, that just can't wait.

Ten hours later, I finish it. I contemplate going to my friend's party, but I know by that stage things will be very messy. I'm too tired and sober for messiness.

The next day, at a recovery session in the pub, everyone looks unwell — except for Loretta and Tim, two die-hard Cats fans, who are grinning as they bask in the glory of their team's ninth premiership. They danced till dawn and shared tequila with strangers in the street. I find out that fans were well behaved at the game, with just 14 arrests in a crowd of nearly 100,000. It's hard to imagine a similar result if Scottish football fans were allowed to drink at matches.

Days later, the premiership cup has barely left the engravers when Carlton & United Breweries release a limited-edition, blue-and-white Geelong-themed slab, with 24 commemorative AFL-endorsed cans wrapped in the triumphant team's photo. Around the same time, Lion release a similar special-edition Tooheys slab in Manly Warringah Sea Eagles colours, celebrating the rugby league team's premiership success. In a country where sport is a national religion, cashing in on that passion is a sure-fire money-spinner.

And it's no longer just the traditional blokey sporting codes that are being propped up by booze. At the start of the year, I visited the Australian Open for the first time in five years. A lot had changed since my last outing. It seemed that for some visitors, tennis was now much further down the list of priorities than getting wasted. As my friend Nat and I stood at the front of a queue outside Margaret Court Arena at 7.00 p.m., a group of boys staggered over. The one at the front was not in good shape: his eyes were glazed over; his once-white T-shirt was smattered with stains. 'We're at the front of the line,' he yelled into his phone, a fug of musty beer breath wafting an unwelcome path towards me.

'Actually, you're not at the front of the line,' I pointed out. 'You've just cut in. The back of the queue is there.' I gestured to the 30 people lined up behind us.

Oblivious, he swayed, shifting the weight of his gangly frame from one foot to the other. The warm evening breeze seemed enough to knock him over. But he was bulletproof. 'We're at the front of the line,' he hollered again. His height gave the illusion of maturity, but he couldn't have been more than 17 — 18 at a stretch. His spotty friends, less vocal but similarly under the influence, looked even younger. They were sunburnt and shit-faced. The steward, trying to manage the growing queue for the match between Ukrainian Illya Marchenko and my fellow countryman and fifth seed Andy Murray, was struggling to control them. Eventually, security moved them on. They loped off, perhaps in search of one more for the road. And they wouldn't have had far to stagger.

There's no shortage of opportunities to buy alcohol at the Australian Open. Don't get me wrong — I don't think we should deny tennis fans the pleasure of a cold beer or a glass of wine in the summer sunshine while watching some of the biggest names in the game take to the court. It's one of the few sporting events that sees tourists from all over the world converge on Melbourne to cheer on their homeland heroes. This carnival atmosphere has earned it the title of the 'friendly' slam. But a shift is taking place. When the over-abundance of alcohol starts to alter the atmosphere and it feels like Melbourne's King Street on a Saturday night, something's wrong. Packs of shirtless young men staggering around, clutching pots of beer and turning the air blue with obscenities, is not a pretty sight.

Judging by the logos and branding hung from every lamppost, flagpole, and awning, Jacob's Creek and Heineken are bigger names at Melbourne Park than Federer and Nadal. The sponsorship of these global brands has no doubt allowed the Open to grow, pouring more cash into the event's coffers and getting more people through the gates, but at what cost? The beer garden has become so enormous that calling it a garden is a bit like calling the *Titanic* a dinghy. On the Thursday night we visited, there was a queue to rival any city nightclub just to get in. Inside, there were bars, deckchairs, live music, and takeaway outlets selling the sort of overpriced, deep-fried food best consumed after several pints; it was an environment engineered to give visitors no reason to leave. Some of the people I spoke with confessed that they hadn't seen one stroke of tennis since arriving at the bar, directly from work. Despite the two giant screens, they couldn't even tell me if home-crowd favourite Sam Stosur had won her match. For these visitors, coming to the tennis was all about drinking.

Organisers have to take some responsibility for reinforcing this association. What used to be called 'Super Saturday' — the biggest day of the tournament's first week, allowing the public the chance to see some of the best players for the cost of a ground pass — has been renamed 'Heineken Saturday'. On the front page of the Australian Open's website, an article in which Heineken was named 13 times appeared to be little more than an advert for the Dutch beer company. Writer Matt Trollope enthused: 'Assigned with the task of writing about Heineken Day, I meandered over to Grand Slam Oval at 15 minutes past noon. The first thing that stood out was the queue. Hundreds deep, it proved that the Heineken Beer Garden was the place to be.'

With my beer goggles removed, I can see the inherent absurdity in the fact that alcohol underpins practically every social pastime that our culture values. It seems as if our enjoyment of the game — whether it's tennis, cricket, rugby, or football — can only be complete by adding alcohol. Having a few drinks as you watch sport can be fun, but it will be a shame if the Australian Open ends up like Melbourne's Spring Racing Carnival — an event now synonymous with epic levels of binge drinking, where the sight of punters passed out, facedown in the Flemington turf, is not uncommon, and thousands of racegoers are lucky to get within 100 metres of a horse.

Drinking is an intrinsic part of our sporting culture. It's tied up with notions of coming of age, male bonding, and community cohesion, particularly in small country towns, where the local sports-club bar is a central meeting point. Run well, sports clubs can be the lifeblood of communities, providing purpose for young people and allowing families to spend time together at the weekends. But there's growing evidence that the link between these clubs and drinking is causing damage. Studies carried out by the Australian Drug Foundation found that almost a third of 13- to 17-year-olds had participated in unsupervised drinking at a sports club. Most were not asked for proof of age. Twenty per cent of 18- to 20-year-olds drank ten or more drinks every time they visited the club. Across members of all ages, more than half drank at hazardous levels on each visit.

This culture of heavy drinking can spill over into violence. In 2009, 37-year-old Nathan Alsop died after being punched in the head by teammate Daniel Singleton at a party to celebrate East Geelong Football Club's grand-final win. Alsop was estimated to have drunk 39 drinks over 13 hours at the team's clubhouse before the altercation. At a later trial, Singleton was acquitted of manslaughter. A week before Alsop's death, New South Wales rugby league fan Geoff Larnach died, after suffering a cardiac arrest and suspected brain damage following an all-day drinking session that started at the Bathurst Panthers Leagues Club. The 27-year-old is believed to have sculled half a bottle of rum to mark the team's season-ending loss. He was described by one of the club's players as their 'number one supporter'.

But what happens if you take grog out of sport? Would, as the alcohol industry claims, grassroots clubs fold? Across Australia, more than 4300 sports clubs have discovered that far from going under after kicking alcohol out of the game, they're thriving. The clubs, all members of the Australian Drug Foundation's Good Sports program, which aims to turn around sport's heavy-drinking culture by promoting a more responsible approach to alcohol, are seeing the benefits, both on-field and off, of reducing the influence of booze in their game. The program was set up in 2000, after Victoria Police asked the ADF for help in reducing the high rates of underage drinking, violence, and drink-driving associated with the boozy culture in community sport. Under the scheme, clubs achieve accreditation for meeting standards around the use and management of alcohol. Measures include banning post-match beers in the dressing room, along with alcoholic raffle prizes and rewards for on-field performance. Sponsorship from pubs or alcohol companies is not accepted. More soft drinks and low-alcohol alternatives are offered at the bar, and meals are served in a bid to attract more families. Club-wide policies that make sure staff, players, and supporters are on board have seen drink-driving, as well as underage and risky drinking, plummet.

At the North Eltham Wanderers Cricket Club in Melbourne's northern suburbs, alcohol sales dropped by 30 per cent when they signed up to Good Sports. But the losses were offset by greater spending in the club canteen, as families previously deterred by the 'boozy boys'-club culture' returned. On-field performance also improved. An analysis of Good Sports clubs earlier this year found that, on average, there were 36 per cent fewer people drinking at risky levels than in clubs not affiliated with the program. Most importantly, many clubs have seen sponsorship dollars grow by getting rid of alcohol sponsors, as organisations previously unwilling to be associated with clubs notorious for heavy drinking have backed the new-look teams. One club has cleaned its image up so much that it's now sponsored by a local church. Perhaps calling last drinks doesn't have to mean game over.

I AM NOT a runner. At least, that's what I've been telling myself for years. Until recently, even ten minutes of road running would leave me wheezing like a two-pack-a-day smoker. But cheered on by my brother, Neil — who, in the last few years, has taken up running with the dedication of a professional athlete — I decided to change that. When I gave up booze, I started going for long runs on the treadmill, increasing my time and speed gradually until I could run five or six kilometres without too much effort. Running in the outside world was a tougher challenge, and I struggled at first. But again, I built up my strength and stamina until I could run on the road for seven or eight kilometres at a time.

Today, I aim to top that. I've entered the ten-kilometre event in the Melbourne Marathon. It's my first-ever race. I'm nervous that I won't finish, or that I'll have to walk part of the way, or that I'll collapse in a heap metres from the finish line.

When my fellow runners Nat and her husband, Gary, pick me up at an ungodly hour, it's still pitch-dark. The roads are quiet. As we drive through the CBD, we see countless young men and women staggering out of nightclubs and strip joints, yelling and swearing, forming queues outside kebab shops and wandering aimlessly in the street. Girls with mascara-streaked faces teeter on shoes with ice-pick heels. Boys, glassy-eyed and incoherent, lope around like injured animals. As we park near the race start line, I bounce out of the car and start stretching in the crisp dawn air. How strange yet satisfying it feels to be on the other side.

I used to laugh at people like us. After my leaving party at The Rose Hotel, Loretta and I and some of the locals ended up at the Tankerville — a 24-hour Fitzroy pokies emporium and bar that can only be tolerated in the early hours of the morning, when you're too wasted to notice the scary-looking dudes at the next table or the neon-blue anti-addict lights in the bathrooms. As we staggered out at 6.00 a.m., making faces at the hippies doing a hot yoga class next door, we spotted some people running on treadmills on the first floor of the gym opposite. We laughed and mimicked their running as if this were the most hilarious thing we'd ever seen. Now Loretta is a yoga teacher, and I'm at the starting line of a ten-kilometre race at seven o'clock on a Sunday morning.

When I start running, I'm mesmerised by the strangely soothing sound of hundreds of feet hitting the tarmac. The noise reverberates in otherwise silent streets that for today are ours alone. I'm happy to discover I'm not the slowest contestant, and I'm even running faster than I was in training. At the three-kilometre mark, a few people have already started to walk, and I vow to myself I will not be one of them. I will finish the game. My brother's pep talk, delivered to me this morning via text message, repeats in my head like a holy sacrament: 'Just remember — PAIN IS TEMPORARY, GLORY IS FOREVER!!!! Persevere, dig deep, enjoy and triumph!!'

There are some funny running styles. Teenage girls in full makeup, with fake tan smudging on stick-thin legs, look awkward as they try to bob along without messing up their hair. One guy runs with his jacket in his hand, while a middle-aged woman wearing a visor and a steely expression appears to be vaulting invisible hurdles. A man wearing board shorts and a singlet looks like he's being chased by the police. I start to get weary around the six-kilometre mark, but find a second wind when I think about all I've achieved in the last ten months. I can do this.

As I reach the seven-kilometre mark on St Kilda Road, there are more spectators lining the street, cheering us on. I feel ten feet tall. I'm smiling. The sun is out, Melbourne has barely woken up, and I'm running towards the MCG, the city's spiritual home. How nice it will be to arrive there, and to feel triumph instead of disappointment.

My body is being pushed to its limits and I realise how far I've come. Would I ever have got here if I hadn't taken a break from drinking? Suddenly, it occurs to me how ridiculous it is that our elite athletes are sponsored by a substance that's simply not conducive to sporting success. How many times have hangovers kept me from the gym, or stopped me from even putting my trainers on and going for a walk?

As I reach the nine-kilometre mark, I'm hurting, but I know I'm home. I can't believe I told myself for so long that I couldn't do this. Maybe now, I can do anything. My legs ache and the balls of my feet are burning, but I power on, sprinting up the hill. I cross the finish line, and it's one of the most exhilarating experiences of my life. The weirdest thing is I don't even feel tired at the end. It takes only a minute or so to catch my breath. I'm so energised by the thrill of finishing, I actually feel like I could keep running. When I receive my race medal, I look at it in awe. I've never been more proud of myself. I am a runner.

November

I CAN'T PUT it off any longer. It was on my list from the start of the year: find love. As much as I've achieved since I gave up drinking, this definitely needs some work. But how do you meet guys if you're not rolling drunk in a bar at 2.00 a.m.? My usual method, falling on top of someone while plastered, is not so easy to pull off when you're in full control of your faculties. Besides, something (perhaps the fact I'm still single) tells me that this strategy wasn't really working.

So I'm left with no choice. Friends tell me everyone's doing it; there's no stigma anymore. It's the modern way for busy singles to meet. But there's something about internet dating that leaves me feeling flat. And more than a wee bit scared. I imagine that the process of dating complete strangers would be excruciating enough with a few drinks to smooth the ride, but the prospect of doing it sober is positively petrifying.

It's not so much that I need a drink to calm my nerves — I know now that poise and self-belief are not measured by alcohol consumption — but that I worry my sobriety will be a barrier to easy conversation in what will already be an awkward situation. Refusing a drink might make guys self-conscious and wary. Maybe that's just something I have to get past if I want to find out how to connect with the opposite sex without being tipsy. I can't remember one alcohol-free first kiss before my break from booze.

I ask my friends for their drunken horror stories and discover that I am far from alone: many of them have used booze as a way to get through the ghastliness of the singles scene. One friend remembers the ignominy of her only attempt at proper, grown-up dating. It was a singles night at a city restaurant, and she and a friend had been slipping tequila shots into their champagne for courage. It worked a bit too well. My friend made a beeline for the most attractive man in the room and shouldered the girl he was talking to out of the way, striking up a flirty conversation. After some chatting, she suggested, 'Shall we try a little kiss now?' This, in her drunken state, seemed like a perfectly reasonable proposal. He said yes. Later, he offered her a lift in his BMW to a bar for more drinks. This meant that he was sober. Mortified by her behaviour, and developing that uniquely intoxicated paranoia that has no connection to reality, she began imagining a future where she was chopped up into pieces and dumped on a waste ground. So she and her friend legged it out of there, leaving their would-be Ivan Milat to train his sights on someone else. The night ended with a vomit in the gutter.

Another friend estimates that she's pashed more than 200 guys in her life, but has experienced only one sober first kiss. Others tell me of boozy travel tales: making sweet love in the laundry room in a Barcelona hostel, or being seduced by a seemingly single neighbour in a London apartment — only to have his girlfriend burst into the bedroom while he was 'heading down south'. One girl recalls working for an investment-banking firm in the United Kingdom and developing a 'massive crush' on the cute Irish boy with whom she shared a desk. 'Cut to a week later at the Christmas party, and I decided if I got just a little tipsy it would be much easier for me to mingle and talk with cute Irish boy. Three hours later, all I remember is begging this poor man to please, please marry me, and then throwing up in his face!'

One friend, who doesn't drink much, says she's been out with several guys who drank heavily, and that proved to be its own challenge. A guy that she'd been on a couple of dates with but hadn't heard from in a few months tried to pick her up in a bar, using the same lines he'd used when they first met. He was smashed, and oblivious to the fact they'd already dated. Yep, it's rough out there.

It makes me wonder how many Australians would be hooking up at all if it weren't for the matchmaking properties of booze. For young people like Beth and her friends, who told me that drinking gives them the confidence to meet guys, alcohol is a key part of sexual attraction. A 2007 survey by the Foundation for Alcohol Research and Education found that 63 per cent of 18- to 24-year-old Australians admitted they'd had a one-night stand while drunk. In the United Kingdom, a 2009 poll of 3000 women found that almost half preferred having sex after a few drinks because it helped them to lose their inhibitions and made them more adventurous in bed. Forty per cent of the 18- to 50-year-olds interviewed said that they were always a bit tipsy before sleeping with a new partner. Six per cent had never had sex sober. Given my experiences and those of my friends, I imagine similar results would be found if Australian women were surveyed.

It seems that drinking to get the romantic juices flowing is an accepted way of finding a mate in modern culture. It's sold to us as an intrinsic part of matchmaking. Dating-coach websites often feature pictures of attractive couples smiling as they share champagne and cocktails. Pubs and nightclubs have been the happy hunting grounds for singles in Australian cities for decades. In rural areas, where isolation makes it harder to meet potential partners, the Bachelor and Spinster Ball is an engrained part of bush tradition. Historically, the events were a way for men and women in farming communities to find a husband or wife, with many travelling long distances to attend the balls. They were big occasions, with a formal dress code and all money raised going to local charities. But over time, they evolved into all-you-can-drink mega-parties — usually sponsored by alcohol companies and local pubs — where getting hammered and having sex was such an integral part of the evening, guests were often given showbags with condoms and lubricant, and offered free breathalyser tests the following morning. The tradition is now waning due to rising costs, the increasing drift of young people from the bush to the city, and tighter regulation around the service of alcohol. But the tradition cemented the inextricable link between drinking and sex in the minds of many Australians.

The idea of alcohol as an aphrodisiac is not a modern notion. The French artists and bohemians of the late 19th century used absinthe as a way to boost their sex drive. These days, champagne has become synonymous with romance and seduction. And there's even some scientific evidence that drinking might help the sparks to fly: a 1994 study in the international journal *Nature* showed that even small amounts of alcohol can enhance a woman's libido, boosting the release of the male sex hormone testosterone in the brain. The same effect was not found in men, and was more pronounced in women who were taking the pill — probably because they had lower testosterone levels than those not taking the oestrogen-based drugs.

It's perhaps not surprising the two should be linked: both alcohol and sex stimulate the release of the chemical dopamine into the brain's reward pathway — essentially, its pleasure centre — sending the signal that the action is pleasurable and worth repeating. If our sexual desire is physiologically altered by alcohol, it might go some way to explaining the thousands of regrettable sexual unions taking place every Friday and Saturday night across the country. But for me, it's rarely about craving the act of sex, and more about satisfying an emotional need. If I drink too much and I'm not in the right headspace to start with, I can really feel the depressive effects of alcohol. It can make me maudlin and sentimental, and will bring any underlying sense of loneliness to the surface. Suddenly, I'm a slave to the urge to be held, or to feel a warm body next to me as I sleep. Add to that the fact that inhibitions and logic usually vanish after about the fourth vodka and soda, turning every knuckle-dragging oaf in the room into Brad Pitt, and you have the perfect storm. At that point, I won't hold out for my knight in shining armour, but — to borrow a phrase from one of my fellow *HSM* bloggers — will be happy to settle for a half-wit wrapped in tin foil. Then, you get him home and it's obvious that, although alcohol may have brought you together, Mother Nature's perverse sense of humour has ensured that it has also caused complete mechanical failure and rendered any chance of sexual satisfaction a physical impossibility. As Shakespeare famously observed, alcohol 'provokes the desire, but it takes away the performance'. Only when you sneak a look at him through one eye the next morning, as he lies there in his chocolate-brown Y-fronts like a pallid monument to regret, do you realise just how drunk you were last night.

I know that my bad decisions can't be explained entirely by alcohol's myopic night vision, but there is some evidence that beer goggles are a scientific phenomenon. In a study conducted by researchers from Bond University, 80 heterosexual men and women aged 18 to 29 were recruited from campus pubs and parties. Three groups were established: really drunk (those with a blood-alcohol concentration of 0.10 per cent to 0.19 per cent — up to four times the legal driving limit); moderately drunk (0.01 per cent to 0.09 per cent); and designated drivers, or people who were sober. The volunteers were shown a series of photos of people of the opposite sex and asked to rate their attractiveness, on a scale of one to ten. Those who were moderately or heavily drunk rated those in the photographs as significantly more attractive than did their sober peers. Getting drunk had turned 'bow to wow'. As the researchers noted, this is a concern, given that previous studies have shown that the more attractive a person is, the more likely their sexual partners are to engage in risky behaviour, such as unprotected sex. But evidence on the beer-goggle effect is inconsistent and inconclusive. In a study published in the *British Journal of Psychology* in 2009, researchers showed 240 men and women, in varying degrees of drunkenness, pictures of other women, and asked them to rate their attractiveness. In this study, drinking alcohol had no effect on how attracted they were to those in the photographs.

With all that in mind, it's probably a good thing that my first crack at internet dating is going to be a sober one. I sit down to set up my online profile, which, I quickly discover, is a unique form of torture. The photograph-selection process involves finding a picture that conveys the delicate balance of friendly but not desperate, serious but not stern, kooky but not weird, and sexy but not slutty. I'm going to need help.

I invite my friends Nat and Mel over, to give me the benefit of their dating wisdom. Nat vetoes one picture because I'm showing too much cleavage. I argue that, given I'm spruiking myself like a house on a real-estate website, this might be the 'appealing north-facing aspect' that gets buyers through the door.

'You don't want those kinds of guys,' she says, deleting the picture, and I'm reminded of just how bad I am at this stuff.

Writing the 'about me' section is another exercise in self-flagellation. How to sell yourself and sound interesting, without coming across as a self-involved twit? We joke that I should write it all in tabloid-newspaper headlines: 'Scottish Chick in Still-Single Shocker' or 'Melbourne's Once-Drunkest Hack on Hunt For Love'. In the end, I settle for what is hopefully a vaguely amusing and informative précis of my passions, hobbies, and life goals.

The part that takes the longest to resolve is the section on drinking habits. There are three options: non-drinker, occasionally/socially, and often. I wonder, much like I do at airport check-ins when they ask if you're carrying any flammable liquids, lighters, or weapons, what kind of person thinks it's a good idea to say yes to the last option, even if it's true. I describe myself as a social drinker, figuring that it's partially correct — given it wasn't that long ago I was the most sociable of drinkers, and I can't see myself ever again drinking in a fashion that could be described as *anti*social. I just can't bring myself to tick the non-drinker box. Even after all I've learned from ten largely fulfilling months without alcohol, I still don't want to be labelled as a teetotaller; the stigma of that is almost worse than the stigma of internet dating. And if I tick the non-drinking box, I worry that I'll attract clean-living fitness freaks, mummy's boys, or Jesus enthusiasts. There is, of course, the chance that I could attract men who, like me, are taking a break from binge drinking, and are interested in self-improvement and a relationship that runs deeper than the bottom of their pint glass, but I'm not willing to take the risk. The world of online dating is massively superficial without adding any additional reasons for men to discount you.

When I hit the button to make my profile go live, it's an unsettling feeling. A friend who's using the same dating site has told me that her sister warned her against it, saying that it was a cyberspace meat market for guys in search of an easy shag. Then she related the tale of a young woman who was kidnapped by a guy she met online and taken to his home, where she discovered that he'd dug a grave in the backyard. She was held captive for two days before being rescued in a police raid. Is this what I'm risking by advertising myself in the most public space imaginable? The site doesn't allow members to use their own names, so at least that's something, but when the system matches me with a reporter from a rival newspaper, and I stumble across my ex-boyfriend's best mate, I realise just how exposed I am.

Each time a new email arrives, a sound like a harp being played goes off. I assume this is meant to signify Cupid at work, but it's quite incongruous with the contact I'm getting from all manner of unsavoury men. Some have instructive names like insatiable7 (presumably insatiable one through six were already taken), rodtherock, romeohadjuliet, and beast. One guy, calling himself Triggerhappy, includes a picture of himself on a plane trying to open the exit doors. It's captioned 'Escape!' Several are holding their crotch (cos the ladies love that shit), while one has posted a montage of scenes of himself frolicking with his dog, including one shot in which they appear to be French-kissing. In one bloke's picture, he's shovelling a foot-long Subway sandwich into his mouth. Another has chosen the seductive 'YOU ARE ALL FULL OF SHIT' as his profile headline. It's every bit as dispiriting as I thought it would be.

But what's even sadder is the desperation and despair evident in some of the profiles. Shattered62 asks, 'Why can't an overweight guy have a cute girlfriend?' There are a lot of broken men out there. I can only imagine what sort of self-esteem problems led Worthalook, WOULDuSETTLE4less, and NotGoodLookingSorry to choose their online names.

I decide to move swiftly past those who are obviously on the rebound, still pining for a lost love, or in need of emotional first-aid. I'm looking for a relationship, not a renovation project. I also bypass anyone who's pictured shirtless and pouting, or lists sex under the 'What I'm Looking For' section, which is a surprisingly large contingent. It's a challenge trying to pick someone that you might click with based on an eight-centimetre square photo, and a few hundred words of what is probably an imaginative sales pitch at best and a complete fantasy at worst. I try not to be superficial, but find myself dismissing any bloke who's wearing a Bintang singlet, thinks that scanning the racing form guide counts as reading, cites *Two and a Half Men* among his favourite television shows, or doesn't know the difference between 'your' and 'you're'. It's a brutal culling process, but it works both ways; I'm rejected by many of the men I contact. My perception of my place in the dating hierarchy takes a battering. Am I destined to be matched with beast or with the sandwich-inhaling guy?

Then I'm contacted by someone who seems normal. His email is fun, flirty, and grammatically sound. He's a self-made businessman and an animal lover. And he's cute — which, let's be honest, is important. As this is my first online date, and essentially a blind date, I arrange to meet him at work. It means that I don't yet have to navigate the awkwardness of refusing a drink in a bar, but I also figure that if he comes to the *Age* cafe, there will be dozens of hacks there to bear witness should he turn out to be a grave-digging sex offender.

When he arrives, I'm impressed. He's well groomed, and dressed in a sharp suit. He has a warm smile, and a calmness to him that's appealing. There's no getting around the weirdness of the situation, though: we are complete strangers trying to make a romantic connection over coffee at 11 o'clock on a Tuesday morning. I don't even know his surname. But we are, at least, fully clothed. I probably already know more about this guy than I ever did about some of the inebriated boneheads that I got naked with hours after falling over them in bars.

My date starts by telling me he's relieved that I look like the pictures on my profile: 'I've had a few bad experiences.' Oh, really; how so? 'Mostly with women lying about their weight. They'd say they were slim when in actual fact they were very large. I've learned that photos taken from the side can be deceiving.' After being misled by five big girls whose pictures had portrayed them otherwise, he went on a sixth date, and when she turned up he took one look at her and said, 'I'm sorry, I have to go.' I'm pretty sure this is what David Brent did to a woman in an episode of *The Office*. It was an awful thing to do, even in a fictitious setting, and I can't help but think less of this man for being so cruel. He says he now uses a microscope to study the online pictures, and we laugh, although I'm not sure he's joking.

We chat about his business and his travels, and how he has changed careers several times already. He seems nervous, but the conversation goes well. I tell him about my job, and somehow, although my strategy had been not to disclose this until at least a second date, we get around to talking about my year without drinking. He doesn't seem immediately horrified, so I explain the situation further. Then he surprises me by telling me that he doesn't drink at all. When I ask why, I'm stunned by his response. He used to drink a lot. He was putting away a bottle of whisky a day from an early age. By the time he was 21, his doctor told him he showed signs of liver cirrhosis. After one massive bender, he was so ill he ended up in a psychiatric ward. After that, he stopped drinking for six months, but he was soon back on the piss. He says he realised that he's the kind of guy who can never stop at one drink. He quit permanently three years ago, and hasn't touched a drop since. I'm amazed that he's sharing this with me on a first date. I don't judge him for it — I know all about the nature of addiction, and I'm impressed by his fortitude — but it's a risk telling a stranger such a personal story. What's even more astounding is that on my first attempt at sober dating, the guy I meet with is a recovering alcoholic. You couldn't make this shit up.

As we make pleasant small talk — about our pets and our heritage and what we do for fun outside of work — I'm trying to figure out if I like him. Am I attracted to him? Sort of. He's cute, but I'm not getting that fire-in-the-engine-room kind of feeling. Do we have a lot in common? Probably not. He seems like a nice guy, barring the fat prejudice, but we're very different. There's no spark, or even the promise of a spark. As we stand up to say our goodbyes, I think, if he asks to see me again, I might give a second date a go just to be sure, but if he doesn't, we'll leave it at that. He doesn't. Perhaps he sensed our difference, too.

But over the next two days I receive a number of texts, emails, and a Facebook friend request, making it clear that he'd like to take things further. He's a tad too keen; I'm indifferent at best. I have to politely let him go. It seems a bit like breaking a business contract. When you meet up sober and you haven't already kissed, swapped bodily fluids, or seen each other tear up the dance floor to 'Highway to Hell', the whole situation seems quite dispassionate. I'm not sure that I handle it very well. And I'm not convinced that dating without alcohol is going to work. I think I need some advice on how to navigate this strange new world.

I contact John Aiken, a 'dating expert' who is also the official relationship psychologist for a leading matchmaking website. In his promotional material, couples talk about how he helped to save their marriage, while singles credit his advice as being the key to breaking their disastrous dating habits. One woman claims that she met her husband just a few months after being coached by John. This sounds like a man who knows his stuff.

When I call John at his Sydney-based business, I tell him about my year without alcohol, and that I want to know how big a part drinking plays in the way singles interact and couples relate. I don't fess up that I'm looking for advice personally. He says having a couple of drinks can put people at ease when they're dating, but there's a fine line between relaxing and losing control. Getting blind drunk on the first date can set up an unhealthy expectation for the relationship, where alcohol becomes the key to the way the couple communicates. For first dates, he says, moderation is non-negotiable: 'It's quite bad when someone's slurring, unsteady on their feet, being loud when they've drunk too much. My advice is always to try and show the other person that you have control over drinking.'

But how much of a negative can alcohol really be in the dating game? Judging from my experiences and those of many of my friends, we might not interact with anyone we were interested in if we were to go completely booze-free, or even just stick to a couple of drinks.

Is alcohol really the reason so many singles are unlucky in love? John tells me that the people he counsels (male and female) are usually in their early to mid thirties, and had thought that by this point in their life they'd be married and have kids, or at least have met their future partner. They're baffled as to why they're having no success. When he questions them, it's often clear that they've been engaging in what he calls 'problem dating behaviours'. They include having sex on the first night or going out with people who are unavailable — those who are married, attached, commitment-shy, or damaged from previous relationships. They also try to push things along too fast by texting or ringing too soon and, too often, writing long emails — generally, showing too much intensity early on. The trigger for these behaviours is frequently alcohol. 'You might start talking about sexually explicit stuff when you're drunk. You might try and get physical with them there at the bar. You could start discussing feelings or the future, or getting too far ahead of yourself, wanting to plan the next date, or to meet their friends, or all that sort of stuff,' John explains. 'You can get caught up in it all, and because alcohol's on board, you lose that filter and you move it far too fast.'

It's as if he's just described the last 15 years of my romantic life. Those things he listed: the text messaging, the physical contact, the clinginess — I've done all of that after a few too many drinks. My alcoholic truth serum has removed my filter and made me act in a way I never would while sober. 'If alcohol is one of the triggers for these behaviours, which it often is, then you need to put some strategies around it,' John suggests. 'So that might be you give yourself a limit in terms of how much you drink. You look at perhaps drinking water in between each drink, or you slow the speed of your drinking down, or you make sure you drink with friends that can keep an eye on how fast you drink. You might also put a time limit on how long you want to stay out before going.'

Once again, just as with Jon Currie, I'm being told to place boundaries around alcohol for my own protection. Getting drunk has been my standard method of meeting and hooking up with guys for as long as I can remember, and to date it has brought me little satisfaction — and often left me feeling empty and cheap, not to mention horribly hung-over. Isn't that what Albert Einstein said was the definition of insanity: doing the same thing over and over, and expecting different results? John says that being sober or drinking moderately allows you to weed out the men who are interested in you for the wrong reasons, rather than adopt the 'scattergun' approach, where you fall for anyone to whom you're moderately attracted and who pays you attention.

'If you're not drinking or if you're a light drinker, it does send a really positive message to members of the opposite sex. But for some reason, people in Australia think it sends the wrong message. They think it means you're a bit boring or maybe a bit uptight, and that's not the case at all. When you drink, you misjudge how loud you are, or you have beer goggles on and start making bad judgements — it's not a great way to try and impress somebody. When a guy meets a woman who's in control of herself, who's good with the banter, and who isn't going to be persuaded by some sort of sleazy one-liner or can give as good as she gets, then that's a turn-on.'

That all sounds good, but my new serene and controlled state has not brought the men flocking. Over the past few months, some guys I've encountered have physically recoiled upon learning that I haven't had a drink since January; flirting comes to an abrupt stop. Their reaction probably says a lot about their intentions, not to mention the extent of their shallowness. But I guess that's John's point. Previously, I may have taken one of those guys home. So how do I change these habits? 'Don't have sex for the first four to six weeks,' he advises me. 'Just take it completely off the table because if a guy's keen he will wait for you. And that's a great way of essentially weeding out any of the players. Then you're focusing on a guy's personality and how you're clicking, rather than, "Are we going to get into the sack?" If you've got a four-week rule of waiting and getting to know the guy, then you're essentially saying, "I'm serious, I'm in it for the long term, and if you're interested in that then go ahead. If not, move on because I want something better."'

Sobriety has certainly helped me to weed out the players. They're so easy to spot they might as well be twirling a pack of Durex round their head and dry-humping the furniture.

John tells me that he's counselled many singles who think alcohol is a magic love potion that will bring them together with the man or woman of their dreams, when in fact over-reliance on it can have disastrous effects.

I ponder this as I head off for my second online date. He's quite different from the last guy: a creative type who works in the arts and loves touring wineries. On this occasion, I arrange to meet him in a bar. It's a Sunday afternoon, which seems like a safe time. When he turns up, he's tall and attractive, but not what I expected. He's got a few prominent tattoos and piercings (which I quite like), and is wearing baggy combat pants hanging down over his arse and exposing his boxer shorts (which I don't like at all). But he's an interesting guy, and chatting to him is easy. He orders a Jameson and dry. He doesn't seem too bothered by my abstinence, but talks a lot about how wasted he's been at recent parties, gigs, and festivals. His laugh is pure Beavis and Butt-head. It's been so long since I've had a drink that maybe all this talk of getting shit-faced is weirder to me than it would be to anyone else, but it just seems sad to hear a 36-year-old man carry on like a teenager.

When he asks me why I'm not drinking, I tell him the story and he quickly shifts into a different gear, saying he knows a lot of people who drink too much. He tells me about an ex-flatmate who used to lock herself in her room and stop paying rent when she went on drinking binges. Sometimes they'd come home to find she'd drunk their beer, filled the bottles up with water, and put them back in the fridge. After she went missing for a few days, they eventually had to break into her room. They found her unconscious on the floor. Her room was littered with bottles. She survived, but, not surprisingly, had to move out.

Why does every guy I meet sober have a horror story about drinking?

I bring the date to an end after a couple of drinks (mine soft, of course) because I know this is not the guy for me. I can tell he's not overly impressed by me either, and as we leave, he pecks me on the cheek and tells me he'll call me when he gets back from an interstate work trip. 'That would be lovely,' I say, knowing that both of us are lying. Sober, I can see that although he's an attractive guy, I'm not attracted to his personality. If I'd been drinking, I probably would have persevered, matching his Jameson and dry with vodka and soda until alcohol made him hotter and that familiar pang of longing for a physical connection took care of the rest. I might not be hooking up with as many guys now I'm sober, but it's so much more empowering to be making choices based on logic and good sense, rather than on alcohol-tainted emotion.

Things become a bit trickier with my third date. This guy is really nice. Within minutes of meeting him for a mid-week after-work drink, I feel completely at ease. We talk about our mutual love of the Hawthorn Football Club, and we share a common taste in music. He is courteous and sweet, and very interested in my job, my writing, and my year without drinking. He's quite handsome, but I'm not instantly attracted to him. When he asks to see me again, I agree to a second date. This time we have dinner, but rather than being grateful that I'm sober, I start wishing I could have a few drinks to move things along more quickly to the kissing stage. Maybe that way, the fuzziness of being tipsy would help me to know whether we had a spark. In the end, although it's clear he's keen, I leave him with just a hug and tell him that I'm too busy working on my book to go on any more dates. It's a cop-out. When he texts me later, saying he'd like to catch up after the book is finished, I have to come clean and admit that I just don't have romantic feelings for him. He's the kind of guy I'd like to watch footy with, but I'm not sure it could go any further than that.

By my fourth date, I'm growing weary. It takes a lot of effort to meet strangers sober, and I decide that this will be my last date until I finish the book. But this guy is great. We hit it off at once, and he shares a love of all the things that make me tick — politics, media, literature, and football. He's passionate and smart and has a great smile. And he makes me laugh. We talk for nearly four hours — two or three times longer than any of my other dates. There's a definite spark. He understands what I'm trying to achieve with my year without booze and the book that will flow from it; he took his own three-month break from drinking recently and gained a lot from it. After having one beer, he tells me I've inspired him, and he starts ordering water. I think this is a good sign. But I'm confused; I'm so unfamiliar with these circumstances. How do I move the evening on from great conversation and subtle flirting to a kiss? If I were a bit drunk, I'd have my hand on his leg by now, or would perhaps employ a light touch of the hand in the small of his back.

Eventually, he tells me he has to go, and as we're standing on the street I'm as nervous as an awkward teenager, wondering what's going to happen next. He leans over and gives me a peck on the cheek, telling me that he'd like to see me again if I'd like to. 'That would be lovely,' I say, meaning it this time. We agree to speak again in a few weeks, when he has returned from a work trip. And we part.

I walk away feeling that something's not quite right. On the tram home, I realise why: this is completely alien to me because I've never done it before. But this is what grown-up dating is like. You go out, you chat, you get to know each other, and over several dates you gradually build up a connection based on mutual respect, trust, and attraction. Until now, I've been unwilling to wait; I've tried to hurry that spark into a six-foot-tall flame of passion by dousing it in alcohol. I thought if I could initiate physical contact — a kiss, a grope, or a shag — I'd know that the guy was interested. Now I can see that all it meant was he was pissed and horny. Even if I never hear from this guy again, tonight will have been worth it for that revelation alone.

WHILE IT MAY be seen as an aphrodisiac or an accompaniment to romance, there's no doubt that alcohol can also help to turn love sour, sometimes in the ugliest of circumstances. John Aiken tells me that, for some of the couples he counsels, problem drinking can ruin the relationship. The glass of wine after work to unwind becomes a bottle, which easily becomes two, morphing into a pattern of heavy drinking during the week, as well as on Friday and Saturday nights. 'You get arguments, you start airing your dirty laundry in public. You can get to the point where you say things you really regret, like, "This isn't going to work out. We're going to get the lawyers in,"' John says. 'Alcohol is a key factor which, if there are problems there already, can fuel the fire. It drops people's inhibitions, and it can lead to aggression and violence, and also just self-destructive behaviour, whether it be flirting outside the relationship, having an affair, engaging in risk-taking behaviour.'

I think about all of the arguments I've had in my relationships, and realise that many of them came during or after a boozy night, when one or both of us had drunk too much. The fights were always verbal, with the occasional slammed door, but for some couples it escalates into more than that. Earlier this year, a Turning Point Alcohol and Drug Centre report revealed that alcohol-related domestic violence in Victoria jumped 15 per cent between 2008 and 2009. In 31 per cent of all cases attended by police, alcohol was a definite factor in the family violence. That's more than 10,300 incidents. Drinking was a suspected factor in a further 5100 cases — a 12 per cent year-on-year increase. Eight out of ten victims were women. Perhaps not surprisingly, many of the incidents occurred during peak drinking times: between 8.00 p.m. Friday and 6.00 a.m. Sunday.

Geoff Munro, head of policy at the Australian Drug Foundation, blames the spike on aggressive supermarket discounting, which has made alcohol available much more cheaply. 'Young people say they find drinks very expensive in nightclubs and bars, so they're often pre-loading with a lot of drinks before they go out. So that may be feeding into more violent and aggressive behaviour in domestic premises.'

Munro, like many of his colleagues in public health, says that the figures support increasing evidence of a correlation between liquor-licence density and alcohol-related incidents. A 2007 study from the National Drug Research Institute showed that every new bottle shop opened in a rural area would lead to 32 assaults, and each new pub in metropolitan locations would spark 17 domestic-violence cases. The study correlated assault figures with the number of 'average-size' bottle shops and pubs to calculate additional annual assaults caused by a new outlet. Pub size was determined by beer sales at each venue. The findings were based on alcohol sales in Western Australia — one of only two states where licensees are legally required to report sales figures. Researchers said that the results were likely to be the tip of the iceberg, as only about one in ten cases of domestic violence is reported. They blamed the increase on the deregulation of the alcohol industry, which led to a proliferation of liquor licences and made alcohol more readily available than ever before. The social consequences of that were evident in increasing violence in the home.

I believe that the industry has an obligation to market and sell its products responsibly, and there's no doubt it should take its share of the blame for the rising social problems that stem from the consumption of those products, but when it comes to stamping out domestic violence, I'm not sure that the answer is simply to take alcohol out of the equation. It's a crime with complex factors at play. When sex, passion, and matters of the heart are involved, people can do dreadful things to one another — drunk or sober. Undoubtedly, throwing alcohol into a volatile relationship is only going to make that worse, but we can't always use drinking as a get-out-of-jail card for our offences, be they emotional or physical.

Research shows that sexual behaviour can be affected even when the drinker has been given a placebo, just as inhibitions and nervousness can be reduced by the mere expectation of alcohol. In a 2001 American study, a group of male undergraduates was played an audiotape of a sexual interaction between two students that resulted in a date rape. They were asked to indicate at four points during the vignette how sexually aroused they thought the woman was, and at what point the man should stop. The men were divided into three groups — those who knew they were drinking alcohol, those who thought it was alcohol but it was actually a placebo, and those who knew they were drinking a placebo. Those who knew or thought they were drinking alcohol took far longer to pinpoint the inappropriateness of the man's behaviour than those in the control group. They also grossly overestimated the woman's level of arousal. The results are alarming, suggesting that, for some people, the belief that they are drunk is enough to excuse the kind of inappropriate and, in some cases, illegal sexual behaviour they otherwise wouldn't engage in.

It makes me shudder, as I think about all the silly things I've done pissed and the dangerous situations I found myself in. At 15, during a night drinking cider in Edinburgh's city centre, two friends and I got into a car with a group of guys we didn't know. We thought we were tough Scottish birds, and that it was all a bit of a lark. The blokes, who must have been in their late teens to early twenties, said they were taking us to a party. We ended up at a flat in Craigmillar, one of the most disadvantaged suburbs in Edinburgh. There was no party. One of the guys climbed in the front window to get into the ground-floor flat; I'm pretty sure it wasn't theirs. They separated us, one locking my friend in the car with him while his two mates took my other friend and me into the flat's communal stairwell. She stayed at ground level, and I was taken up two flights of stairs.

By then, we all knew we'd made a big mistake. The guy started kissing me, and I was too scared to resist. He held my wrist behind my head with one hand and, with the other, yanked down my underwear and began groping me roughly. His full weight was on me, pinning me to the concrete steps. I struggled, telling him to stop. I could hear my friend downstairs doing the same. I yelled out to her and somehow managed to push him off me. Crying, we ran into the street and found our friend in the car trying to fend off the third guy. He opened the door and let her out. They were angry, branding us 'fucking prick-teasing slags'; yet somehow we ended up back in the car and they drove us to my neighbourhood, dropping us a few streets from my house — a perverse act of chivalry from would-be rapists. The three of us ran from the car sobbing.

Twenty years have passed since that night, but the dangers for women when they're drinking remain ever present. When I pick up that hot 20-something in a club, I see it as harmless fun, something to tell my mates about the next day: 'The old bird's still got it.' But with the clarity of sobriety, I can see that taking home men you don't know when you're blind drunk and live alone is unwise, to say the least.

While figures are grey, given that it's hard to determine whether drinking was the direct cause, an estimated 1000 people are victims of drug- or alcohol-related sexual assaults each year. And that's just the ones who report it. Police believe that increasing numbers of women are having their drinks spiked — although, again, figures are hard to pinpoint, as women often don't report or remember the incident. Of course, the blame for sexual violence should never fall on the victim.

Suddenly, sober dating doesn't seem such a silly concept; if nothing else, it's safer.

I'M OFF TO celebrate a happier romantic union: my friend and former flatmate Lucy is getting married. She and fiancé Shanan are well matched, and deeply in love. I couldn't be happier for them. But it's my first sober wedding, and I'm nervous. I'm reminded of how Nick, my teetotaller friend, warned me that 'weddings are the worst' when it comes to having to justify your sobriety.

When I arrive at the reception centre, there are people milling around on the lawn, where the ceremony will take place, but no sign yet of bride or groom. There are a few couples and groups chatting, but I head straight towards a guy who, like me, has arrived alone and looks awkward. I introduce myself, and he reciprocates warmly. He seems like a good guy — and cute, too. Somehow we get around to talking about his most recent holiday, a ten-day trip to Las Vegas. He gambled away $2000. My jaw drops. He says that this was less than what he'd budgeted to lose, and that he made up for it by drinking $200 of alcohol a day in the open-bar deal at the casinos. After so long without a drink, I can't begin to imagine how anyone could consume that much booze in one day.

The ceremony is beautiful, and Lucy, a former model, looks stunning. Afterwards, we head to the bar, and I find myself wondering how much I'd drink today under normal circumstances — a free bar and a room full of people I've never met before would probably merit at least a couple of drinks an hour. Instead, I order orange juice, which I ask to be served in a champagne glass. I'm sick of having to drink my soft drinks out of ugly plastic tumblers.

Apart from Lucy and Shanan, the only person I know today is my other former flatmate, Oliver. At dinner, I'm seated next to him, and he helpfully announces to the whole table that I'm not drinking. I'm asked if I'm pregnant. I say no. Oliver tells them that I'm writing a book about my booze-free year. There are a few astonished faces. A guy sitting opposite me pipes up, 'That would be a really short book. Fucking boring. The end.' I laugh politely, but secretly I want to stab him in the eye with my entree fork. He says that stopping drinking would be easy in winter, but impossible during Melbourne's Spring Racing Carnival: 'You can't not drink at the races. You just can't.' This, it seems, is an indisputable fact. He tells me how he stopped drinking for three months a few years ago, and every day of it was so boring that he'd never do it again. He doesn't appear to see the irony in the fact that with a beer in his hand, he's the most boring man alive.

There's a half-filled champagne flute in front of each of us for the toast. The racing fan tells me that I have to drink for the toast, even if it's just a sip. Across the table, another guy nods gravely, explaining, 'It's the toast. You have to.' Again, I smile, and hope they'll stop staring soon. When Lucy's dad raises his champagne glass to the bride and groom, I raise my orange juice. It's not a popular move. They look at me as if I've cursed the marriage.

Later, when the DJ starts, I realise I'm much better at dancing sober than I was 11 months ago. Busting a move with strangers is a new one, but I get into it, remembering that weddings are the natural home of bad dancing. I am by no means the worst dancer here. It turns out to be a lovely evening, which — apart from the awkward toast situation — is far less uncomfortable than I expected. I flirt with the Las Vegas guy and he flirts back. We dance, and chat about our reading habits, our families, and our love of sport. It seems there's some mutual attraction. But after a lull in the conversation, he gets up abruptly and says he's going to 'hang out with the boys' outside. He doesn't invite me. I laugh as he wanders off. If I'd been drinking, I might have pursued him; I'd have excused his rude behaviour and found a way to make him mine. Sober, I don't care enough to bother. Instead, I return to the dance floor with the bride and enjoy being with her, smiling as I share a moment in the best day of her life. I might be going home alone tonight, but I leave with happy memories, and my dignity intact.

December

THIS COULD BE the toughest month so far. So many parties. I don't want to be a spectator this Christmas, but I wonder if it's possible to be full of festive cheer without the festive beer. It's hard to resist a drink when the weather's warming up — albeit sporadically, in that uniquely Melbourne fashion that sees you digging the electric blanket out of the back of the cupboard the day after you swapped it for a fan. When it's 28 degrees at 6.00 p.m., a knock-off drink in the sunshine seems wholly appropriate. But then I look back to last December, and my desire to crack open a cold one fades. I remember that New Year's Day hangover as if it were yesterday: I can still taste the foul blend of tequila, Baileys, and pale ale; the dull throb around my temples and the stabbing behind my eyes are as real now as they were then. Some memories are relived so large it feels as if they could swallow you whole.

I don't want to go back there. As nervous as I am about a sober party season, I'm more nervous about what will happen when it's over. This year has gone so fast. I worry that, come January, I'll have a sip of beer and before long I'll be back where I started — the health reporter writing about binge drinking and then writing herself off. Being drunk doesn't worry me; it's the fear that it could become a regular pattern again. Moderation is my holy grail, but I'm just not sure it's in me. When I gave up smoking, I learned that I'm not good at doing things by halves. One night in the pub, two years since I'd had my last cigarette, I gave myself permission to have a few puffs, and it tasted good. So I decided I'd be one of those annoying social smokers, who bums cigarettes from friends at parties but never gets hooked. A few months down the track, I was back to two packs a week. I had to quit all over again. I either smoke or I don't — they seem to be my choices. My chocolate habit's the same: once the packet's open, there's no stopping me. Why would drinking be any different?

My first test is an annual get-together of friends, which is traditionally a marathon boozing session. This was the Christmas party that last year started at midday Sunday and rolled on till 5.00 a.m. Monday. This year, festivities start at 5.00 p.m. — we must be getting sensible in our old age. But it's not just about drinking; there's also a feast of food. Each guest (about 25 of us this year) is given prior instruction on what to bring, so the spread is phenomenal: there are platters of canapés; a carvery of roast lamb, pork, and chicken; roasted veggies; prawns; a smorgasbord of salads; and a range of delicious desserts. It's all served on tables joined together to form one huge banquet, decked out in festive paraphernalia and set up in the driveway next to our friends' Northcote townhouse. The evening passes quickly and is heaps of fun. There's one brief moment of panic, when I pick up my glass of Diet Coke and realise a split second before the liquid touches my lips that it is in fact red wine. How devastated I'd be if I inadvertently fell off the wagon just weeks before the end of my alcohol-free year.

I dance so much I get sweaty and require continuous hydration. Usually I'd reach for another beer. This year it's water, and I still feel parched. No wonder I used to get so drunk. I don't really miss booze on this occasion, but I do note that time seems to pass more slowly. Pissed, I floated from person to person, dropping out of one conversation and into the next in a seamless way. Sober, I still mingle, but my movements are more deliberate: there's no gliding from one interaction to another; it's conscious and considered and executed in blunt, staccato moves. It's tiring. What's really interesting is the way Loretta — who this time last year was fresh out of an Indian ashram and bewildered by the drunken shenanigans around her — has re-embraced the group dynamic with gusto. Last year's quiet observer is this year's party girl. I wonder if that will be me a year from now.

I leave just after midnight. I've been to enough parties sober by now to know that from this point on, a time of night I've come to think of as the witching hour, the law of diminishing returns is in play. The longer you stay at a party when everyone's shit-faced and you're sober, the less fulfilling it is; the language of sobriety no longer makes sense to the intoxicated, and vice versa. After nearly a year off the booze, I can pinpoint the exact moment when a night goes awry: I can pick up on the throwaway comment that sparks an argument, the playful nudge that's more of a shove, the lingering look that leads to a morning of regret. The next day, when everyone's puzzling over how a convivial evening turned into a shit-fight, I have the answers. But I've learned to keep them to myself. Some things are best left forgotten.

I leave the party glad that I won't be hung-over tomorrow. There will be no remorseful realisations. But the insecure part of me, even after a year of living without alcohol, worries about being the odd one out. That's something I've been unable to shake — that sense that you're not fully part of the group if you bail early. The next day, over lunch or a pub recovery session, people laugh and swap stories from the tailend of the party and you've got nothing to say. The things you do recall, people would rather not remember.

This is the first party of the season. From here, my Facebook feed starts to fill up with friends posting pictures of themselves wearing Santa hats and drinking champagne. There are endless discussions about aching livers, the horrendousness of hangovers, and the best way to cure them. Australians tend to favour a greasy fry-up and Bloody Marys, whereas my Scottish friends recommend packets of crisps and bottles of Irn-Bru. The Christmas spirit is so abundant, some people have two or three parties in one day. I meet one friend for lunch at the end of a big week, and she's so exhausted she looks like she's hanging on by her fingertips. The festive season is a marathon, not a sprint.

At work, management put out the annual Christmas-party warning, reminding us that the standards of the workplace are to be maintained at all social functions associated with Fairfax Media. I'm not sure when they last visited our newsroom, but they might want to rephrase that — unless they want us all to swear like wharfies and crack jokes that would make a sailor blush. The email also warns that harassment, offensive or inconsiderate behaviour, and excessive alcohol consumption — the hallmarks of any good Christmas party — are all off-limits. It's perhaps understandable that our bosses want to save us from ourselves: December is a month of mayhem. The weather's warming up, work finishes, and holidays begin, making it one of the busiest times of the year for emergency services. The last working day before Christmas marks the start of a huge spike in alcohol-related problems, with a 50 per cent increase in ambulance callouts for alcohol intoxication on that day alone. New Year's Eve is the same. Too much festive spirit can ruin even the best party.

On the day of the *Sunday Age* party, some colleagues ask if I'll drink. They suggest that a big night on the piss would be good for the dramatic arc of my book's narrative, and offer to assist me in my relapse. I can't think of anything more absurd or disappointing than getting this far only to get drunk two weeks before the end. Several colleagues joke that it just won't be the same without the seasonal Starkers outburst. One workmate remarks, 'You're like a fat comedian who loses lots of weight. You're just not as interesting.'

I vow to challenge this perception at the party and, after a couple of cranberry and sodas, I front my editor, who's been sitting in a corner talking to the same two staff members for an hour, and demand that she mingle. It's a rare chance for her to spend time with our many talented freelancers, and she should get out there and press the flesh. She's surprisingly acquiescent, and starts to work the room.

As the evening progresses, I make more verbal gaffes, blurting out opinions perhaps best kept to myself, and I realise anew that it's not alcohol that makes me tactless; it's just my personality.

But in a sign that she forgives my forthrightness, my editor tells me that she thinks it's an extraordinary achievement to have gone so long without a drink, one that she confesses she doubts she could match. Even Cam, the man who told me my book about not drinking could be titled 'My Year With No Mates', is full of praise. 'Well done, Starkers. That's a fucking monster effort,' he says, as he clinks my lemon, lime, and bitters with his beer. I examine the comment for his trademark sarcasm, but find none. It makes me pause to reflect. A whole year without alcohol — it's really something. In recognition of this, in the annual staff awards I receive the Sober as a ... Journalist Award for 'being off the booze for over a year, despite occupational hazard'. It's quite a turnaround from last year's inaugural Jill Stark Drinking Award.

I leave the party at 11.00 p.m., feeling satisfied that I've had a good night but with the niggling sense I might be missing out on some fun. In the morning I wake up feeling ever so slightly hung-over, which is odd, given that I drank soft drinks and water all night. But I have all the signs: a dry mouth and a slight headache, and I'm very tired. Perhaps it was the cigarette smoke at the rooftop bar, or maybe I overdosed on sugary soft drinks. It could be a phantom hangover — the memory of Christmas parties past. Last year, I managed four hours' sleep between leaving the after-party pub session and rocking up to work, and previous years were no different. Maybe my body is so used to waking up in a state of wretched disrepair after this event, it has reacted accordingly. Whatever the reason, it's as if my body's reminding me of what I haven't missed over the last 12 months. Those hangovers, with the exhaustion, the scratchy throat, the craving for carbs, and the heightened feelings of melancholy and lethargy, were so debilitating. I'm not sure the reward I got from a few beers was worth enduring those mornings-after.

I ARRIVE EARLY and sit at a picnic table in a courtyard near the emergency department. A man wearing shorts and a singlet is smoking a cigarette and shuffling slowly towards the cafe behind me, wheeling a drip beside him. He looks at me and I offer a smile; he casts his eyes to the ground. I wonder what he's in for. It's been six months since I was last here. When I came to meet Jon Currie at St Vincent's for an interview that evolved into a clinical diagnosis, I was wrapped up in a scarf and a thick coat.

A warm breeze gains momentum, picking up napkins and random detritus, and scattering them across the courtyard. My heart flutters in unison. It's taken so long to arrange these brain scans that I thought it would never happen. Part of me was glad. But when I got the email, it became real. I had to read it twice before it sank in. It came from a neuroimaging scientist at St Vincent's Centre for Clinical Neurosciences and Neurological Research. He said the scan would involve 'high-resolution structural images, along with diffusion-weighted imaging, allowing us to generate 3D images of the white-matter tracts of the brain'. I wasn't entirely sure what it meant, but it sounded serious. Now I'm at the hospital, I'm terrified by what these images will show.

I make my way from the courtyard to the neuroimaging department next door. When I arrive, the front door is locked. It's Saturday. I press a buzzer and tell the voice that answers I'm here for an MRI. Suddenly, I am a sick person.

The MRI centre is in the basement. I can hear machines whirring, and the distant sound of an alarm. Other than that, it's eerily quiet. The reception area is decked out in tinsel and two fake Christmas trees, but nothing about this place feels festive. The receptionist takes an inordinate amount of time to find me on the system. I wonder if I've been filed under a different category from all the genuinely sick people — perhaps there's a separate sub-section for time-wasting binge drinkers.

I sit down on a squeaky blue chair. There are two other women in the waiting room, both in their sixties. When it's my turn, a nurse, Milly, ushers me down a long corridor into the MRI area, and we sit down at a desk. She pulls out a form, recording my weight and allergies. She asks if I could be pregnant, and if I have a pacemaker or any body piercings. No. Then she reels off a list of conditions I must disclose. Diabetes? No. Epilepsy? No. Heart disease? No. Any liver damage? I pause. She looks up, raising one eyebrow. 'Not that I know of,' I reply in a whisper.

'So we're scanning your brain today?' she says, the way a hairdresser might discuss options ahead of a cut and colour.

'Yes, please,' I reply, my tone unintentionally eager.

I'm led into a changing room, where I take off all my clothes except my undies, and put on royal-blue hospital scrubs. As I fold my singlet and skirt and place them neatly in a metal locker, I wonder what Milly thinks of me. Does she know why my brain is about to be scrutinised from every conceivable angle? How many alcoholics does she see here? Or is it mostly people with brain tumours? Oh my God. What if they find a brain tumour? How many patients leave this department with life-changing, or life-ending, news? I close the locker door and lean my head against it. Slow, deep breaths.

When I come out, I'm met by the MRI technician. She tells me her name, and I instantly forget it because at the same moment I spot over her shoulder the machine I'm going to spend the next

45 minutes trapped inside. It's just as imposing as it looks in the hospital shows on television. It screams sickness. I lie down on what I suppose is a bed of sorts, my feet slightly raised. She tells me that she's going to put a cap on my head — it's a bit like a bike helmet. I must lie completely still. If I have an itch, I can't scratch it. She lays a blanket over me and inserts foam earplugs in my ears. 'The machine is very loud and for one of the scans, it will vibrate quite a bit. Don't worry, that's normal,' she tells me, her voice sounding as if we're underwater.

Lying motionless under my blanket, I feel like a corpse wrapped in a shroud. She moves two padded plates to the side of each temple, securing my head in a gentle vice. The bed moves backwards into the machine as I see her, in the mirror above me, leave the room and take up a position behind a monitor in the viewing area next door. She watches me through the glass.

When it starts, the noise is frightening. A loud and angry buzzer sounds again and again. So much for my plan to meditate my way through this. The next one is lower, like a foghorn, and slower, but just as loud. After a while, I start to get pins and needles in my hands, wrists, and forearms. They're never still for this long. The last noise is the worst. It's a siren, fast-paced, and similar to the sound accompanying the green man on a pedestrian crossing, only two octaves higher and twice the speed.

After a few minutes, the vibrations start. First they're around my head, and then my temples, and then underneath me. They are violent. The machine shudders as if the green man were wielding a pneumatic drill. I really want this to stop, but I lie here. Still.

When it's over, the bed moves out of the machine and I jump up. The blood rushes to my head and I sway. I can only imagine how much more terrifying that experience would be if you knew that the results of the scan could alter the course of your life. I hope that's not the case for me.

The whole experience is finished in just over an hour. As I leave, I go past the waiting room and see a man in a baseball cap and shorts, his limbs limp and wasted. He's slumped forward in one of the blue chairs, snoring loudly. Fellow patients flick through gossip mags and fumble with their phones as though he were no more than an apparition, but I can't stop staring. This emaciated man, whose body has defied him, seems portentous. Is he my Ghost of Christmas Yet to Come?

I'M INVITED TO a friend's Christmas cocktail party. It's a house party, but quite a special event: all-you-can-drink beer, wine, and champers, plus a different cocktail served on the hour every hour, with accompanying canapés cooked by an apprentice chef from one of Melbourne's most famous fine-dining restaurants. I'm a bit bummed that I can't enjoy the cocktails, but our hostess Mari-Claire kindly offers to have her resident mixologist whip me up matching mocktails. At least I'll look like I'm drinking the same exotic concoctions as the other guests.

When we arrive late on Sunday afternoon, everyone is dressed up and looks fabulous. It's a great atmosphere. The other guests start off with beers and champagne, while I go with water.

The first cocktail is served. It's a peach Bellini. Mari-Claire tells me my non-alcoholic equivalent is on its way and heads back into the kitchen. A few minutes later, she proudly hand-delivers my drink. I'm so used to being the odd one out that there's something quite thrilling about being given a champagne coupe, frothy-pink and sparkling, like all the others. I admire it for a couple of seconds, and take a swig. As it hits the back of my throat, there's a sharpness that I recognise instantly. In that split-second, something snaps. I feel a surge in my brain like electricity rushing through a powerline. It's alcohol.

Thoughts and emotions tumble over one another in my head.

Suddenly, I'm consumed with the possibility of getting drunk. Who would know? I'm certain it's alcohol, but I tell myself that maybe it's just a bitter-tasting mixer, such as tonic. Better take another sip. I get another surge of electricity. I can see myself knocking back beers and partying into the next morning. The buzz is exhilarating.

Then, I realise what's just happened. Less than two weeks to go, and I've failed. Can I really say I went a year without alcohol after this? Tears well as I turn to Loretta and hand her my glass. 'Taste that. Is it alcohol?' I watch her as she tastes and nods. I'm devastated. She puts a hand on my shoulder and tells me that it's okay, it was two sips and it doesn't count. I didn't know it was alcohol. Mari-Claire is hugely apologetic. This was no sabotage — it was a genuine stuff-up. She makes me a new one, and this time the champagne is replaced with soda water, as per the original plan.

For the next hour, I battle a voice in my head that says, 'Fuck it. You might as well get drunk.' I prevail and enjoy the rest of my night sober, trying not to dwell on the mishap. As a consolation prize, I smoke a few of the joints being passed around, knowing that this is a bad idea but doing it anyway. Then I smoke a few more.

I get chatting to a girl I vaguely recognise, but have never formally met. People are limbo-dancing on concrete in the driveway. The ground is getting wet and slippery as rain cascades over the side of the tin roof, covering the makeshift dance floor. I tell the girl that someone's going to end up on their back. She replies, 'It'll be nothing compared to the fall you took last year.' I have no idea what she's talking about. She tells me that at one of these Christmas parties last year, I was dancing on a kitchen floor slippery with beer when my legs went from under me and I flew into the air, landing on my back with such an impact that there were real concerns I might have broken something. That's how she recognised me. I'm *that* girl. 'The noise when you hit the floor was unbelievable. We were amazed you just got back up and kept dancing,' she says, smiling. I laugh, nodding to my water bottle and remarking on how different things are this year. Quietly, I'm troubled that my brain has erased all memory of this event. Landing flat on my back on a cold, hard dance floor is exactly what I did on my 25th birthday, ten years ago. Now seems a good time to leave.

Only when I get in my car to drive home do I realise how stoned I am. It's lashing down rain. I'm doing about 40 kilometres in an 80-kilometre zone, gripping the steering wheel like a 90-year-old grandmother. When I reach an intersection I don't recognise, I take a wrong turn and end up doing laps in a McDonald's car park, unable to find the exit. I feel like I'm trapped in an Escher painting. My brain starts to eat itself. How the fuck do I get out of this car park?

After several more laps and a string of expletives, I finally find the road home. My heart is pounding. I'm an idiot for driving in this state. How horribly ironic it would be to go nearly a whole year without drinking, only to be arrested for driving while stoned ten days before the finish line. When I pull into my car park, relief floods my muscles and leaves me limp. I kiss the steering wheel and, despite more than three decades of devout atheism, cross myself.

Lying in bed, I'm exhausted, but I can't sleep. That sip of alcohol stays with me. I'm worried about the way I reacted when the champagne passed my lips — that surge of electricity. It felt so wrong, and yet so right.

TWO DAYS LATER, I turn up to a scheduled appointment with Jon Currie to discuss the results of my brain scans and to take more tests. I arrive at his Fitzroy addiction clinic, fittingly housed in an old building that used to be a pub and still has the name, Devonshire Arms Hotel, inscribed in stone above the door.

He shows me into his office. On his computer screen is a bluish image of my brain, taken from above, on a black background. It's very weird to see my scalp exposed like that, my brain sitting behind what looks like two white golf balls, but are actually my eyes. In another image, my profile is visible — my nose, lips, and chin — just as in a photograph, except that I've been sliced in half, I have no hair, and you can see my spinal cord running up to my brain. He points to the grey matter of my brain and says that we're looking for shrinkage in these areas. He's also looking for damage in the white tracts that run between the grey matter like fat, wiggly worms. These are the cables that transfer information. I'm staring at the screen, but I have no idea what's bad and what's good. Is it damaged or not?

After an insufferably long silence, he says quietly, 'This looks like a normal, happy brain.' For the first time, Jon's telling me something that doesn't make me feel nauseated. 'The good thing is you've emerged from your 12 months with a normal, healthy brain. What we don't know is whether it was a normal, healthy brain 12 months ago.'

I'm so relieved. He tells me there's evidence to show that some structural damage in white matter caused by drinking can improve over time, if you catch it early. It would have been fascinating to know if my brain was in a state of disrepair at the start of the year and my break from booze has healed it. We can only speculate on whether half a lifetime of binge drinking had taken its toll. But I remember how heavy my head felt on those Saturday mornings at work, when my Friday-night partying made everything so slow and laborious. It felt as if my brain wasn't functioning properly. I don't need definitive evidence that it was damaged to know that I don't want to feel that way again.

Jon tells me it's great that there's no obvious large-scale damage or shrinkage in my brain. But these MRI scans only look at structural damage; how well my brain actually functions is another story altogether. Now, I have to sit a battery of neurocognitive tests, which will go some way to finding out whether more subtle damage has occurred. I spend an hour in front of a laptop computer with one of his research assistants, doing tests that literally make my brain hurt.

They're touch-screen exercises designed to test memory, attention, cognitive flexibility, and planning and problem-solving skills.

The first test is fairly simple. Two boxes containing a number of circles flash up, and I have to click on the box with the smallest circle. On this, I score above-average, with results that are better than 80 to 95 per cent of people in my age group (24 to 39), meaning that my capacity for sustained attention is good. In a more challenging exercise, I have to watch numbers scrolling quickly and continuously. I must click a button when I recognise three pre-determined sequences: 2, 4, 6; 4, 6, 8; and 3, 5, 7. On this, I also score highly. In a test of my immediate memory I'm below average, with results better than only 15 to 20 per cent of the population. This doesn't surprise me at all. But the one that gives me the most difficulty involves replicating a pattern of three coloured circles in the least number of moves, abiding by rules that limit the way the circles can be moved. I successfully complete five out of a possible 13 in the allotted time, giving me a score that is well below average, better than only 5 per cent of the population.

When I ask Jon what these test results show, he says that it may indicate deficits in my memory and my planning skills. 'You struggled quite a bit with those tests, which was interesting. Here's a high-IQ person, and although you would not make a diagnosis off that one test, it does suggest you have some trouble with those forward-planning, high-level things. It means multi-tasking, making rapid parallel decisions, and also, in a sense, learning from your mistakes. So it's making complex decisions from complex information, and you may struggle with that.' This may explain my woeful sense of direction, complete inability to read a map, and tendency to pursue the same loser guys who always disappoint me.

He asks me about my short-term memory. I tell him it's poor, to the point that if I didn't use shorthand or a tape recorder I'd struggle to remember many details of an interview an hour after

I've conducted it. I can read a book and quickly forget the plotlines or characters, even if I loved it. He says that the brain's prefrontal cortex is responsible for short-term memory, and it's common to see people who have been binge drinking from an early age with subtle impairment in this area. The prefrontal cortex also controls inhibition — again, commonly impaired in chronic binge-drinkers. I tell him about my short temper, my infamous truth-telling sessions, and my unfortunate habit of blurting out my unfiltered opinions. This habit has not ceased since I stopped drinking.

'Looking at these results and your history, you'd have to ask yourself, how much of that is slightly impaired impulse control, or difficulty in putting the brakes on things?' he says. 'It may just be personality, so you can't necessarily say you drank and therefore you have this, but it might be that you would have been slightly better at this, slightly better at that, slightly less off the handle. But with that history of binge drinking, you may have locked those pathways into always craving more alcohol.'

Given my history of depression and anxiety, which may or may not have been triggered by early binge drinking, Jon says that returning to a pattern of regular heavy drinking would be inadvisable. 'There's no doubt that, post-drinking, you do get quite major surges of depression in the period where you don't drink. We've just done a study looking at people who didn't drink at all versus people who drank [at] low, medium, and high levels — which is two drinks a day, six drinks a day, and ten drinks a day. We looked at what their brains looked like when they were drinking, and what they looked like after one day of not drinking. Even those with low levels of drinking had changes in the chemical structure of the brain, and they had withdrawal patterns one day after stopping. In other words, their excitatory system and inhibitory systems were not normal. So just the regular exposure can mean that you are struggling with a brain that isn't functioning completely normally.'

My real worry is what just happened at the weekend: two sips of champagne that led to a sudden desire to get drunk. One of my friends told me that I was reading too much into it, and I was just excited at the novelty after so long without alcohol. I suspect that Jon will have a different take on it. He does. 'Isn't it fascinating that it's still there? A year later, almost to the day, and you still could have happily got really drunk. These pathways are still significantly locked in. That's a very salutary experience you've just had. It shows that this sensory-memory pathway for drinking is well and truly set up in your brain. It's a conditioned reflex, and you felt excitement, the reward — that's exactly what gamblers feel. It suggests there's a moderate propensity to go on and get in trouble; it's certainly indicative of increased risk. If you're getting that degree of interest in your brain, then that suggests that it would be a warning sign. You may be one of these people who quickly clicks back into it.'

I tell him about getting stoned at the party. It was the first time since Easter, when I had a few puffs and felt dreadful, that I'd smoked a joint. He says that resorting to it as a consolation for not letting myself get pissed may be my pleasure-seeking brain's attempt to substitute one substance for another.

So where do I go from here? The results of these tests aren't as definitive as I'd have liked. I almost feel as if I need to start drinking again to know if I can drink moderately. He says that if I do, I should do it with a 'life jacket': someone who can monitor my drinking in a dispassionate way; not a friend who might tell me what I want to hear, but someone impartial. This is what he does with many patients who return to controlled drinking. They keep a diary of their consumption, and every two months they visit him to discuss their progress. 'If you're reasonably accurate about the record of what you're doing, then you'll get a guide as to whether it seems to be spiralling out of control. That's something that otherwise you might kid yourself and not be truthful about, and then find in a year or so you've gone very quickly backwards. If that happens, I would think you'd need to seriously think about not drinking.'

At home that night, I find this hard to process. When I started this ride, there was no doubt in my mind that I'd go back to drinking when the year was up. Now, I'm not sure. The test results were inconclusive, but the suggestion that some of my shortcomings might not be innate personality traits but self-inflicted scars is enough to make me pause to consider what drinking is really worth. It's clear that the older I get, the less I am able to cope with these massive weekend binges. If I go back to the same pattern, what will my brain function be like ten years from now? Then again, I'm so much more conscious of my moods, my emotions, and my reasons for drinking that I'd like to think I could drink in a mindful way, and not let alcohol dictate how my night ends up.

But then, I think about the cocktail party. What would I have done if that party had taken place two weeks from now? Sometimes freedom is a burden. Once my year's up, there will be no self-imposed abstinence or public expectation to make the decision for me. If I indulge in the occasional blowout, how rapidly would I go back to getting pissed, even when I don't feel like it? Would I be stumbling home at 5.00 a.m. when I meant to leave the party four hours earlier? I can now see why Will talks about degrees of addiction. I don't think I'm an alcoholic. And all of the things those test results suggested may be natural character traits that would have been there regardless of whether I was a big drinker. But I do worry that booze has more control over me than I'm comfortable with. Why else would the thought of drinking again worry me so much?

The thoughts chatter on in my head, and I try to settle them with deep breathing. But it's a hot night, and I can't sleep. The Christmas-party season is in full swing: outside my apartment, people are yelling and beeping horns; groups of guys are leering out of car windows. Later, I'm woken by an awful spluttering noise and think that my cat must be choking on a hairball. I race to the living room, but he's curled up on the couch asleep. The noise is coming from outside. I peer through the blinds and see a woman about my age on her knees, vomiting in the gutter. Two friends standing over her are eating hot chips and laughing. Nothing says 'Merry Christmas' quite like a stranger chundering outside your bedroom window at two o'clock on a Wednesday morning.

It reminds me of an article I read this week by Ruby Rose, the model and MTV presenter, about her 90-day break from booze. Her decision to quit drinking came when she threw up on American pop starlet Katy Perry, after they crashed a high-school formal. The 25-year-old said sobriety had taught her that being pissed isn't sexy; she realised that red eyes, smudged lipstick, and slurred speech are not attractive. I guess it just goes to show that whether you're an average Joe spewing in a suburban gutter or a smoking-hot celebrity vomiting on an international superstar, alcohol will happily take you there.

I can't see myself chucking my guts up in a gutter any time soon, but I do worry that by welcoming booze back into my life, my days of *carpe diem* will be gone. I'll be back to lethargy and excuses. Without alcohol, I've been more fearless than I have in years.

Earlier this month, the music school where I've been taking singing lessons had an end-of-term concert. In a busy bar in front of dozens of people, students of all ages got up and faced their fears. It was an incredibly moving experience to see people who'd never performed in public before stand in front of the mike and realise a dream. The youngest was 12, and the oldest 65. It taught me that you're never too old to achieve your goals. But at the same time, it made me realise that I don't want to wait. I've got the confidence and motivation now, so I shouldn't let anything stop me. When it was my turn to sing, my friends Loretta, Kath, and Lili cheering me on, my nerves disappeared, and I was completely absorbed in that exquisite moment. I was wearing my undies on the outside, and it felt fantastic.

I'M HEADING TO Sydney for Christmas with Loretta and her family. Then we'll drive back down the coast, to a New Year's Eve party at a friend's beachfront property along the Great Ocean Road. I can't wait to take a road trip and have some time away.

People keep asking how I'll survive the holidays without drinking. It's fairly simple — I just won't drink. I've been doing it for 51 weeks, so one more will be easy. True, for most of my adult life I've had a drink on Christmas Day. But with all that rich food, free-flowing wine, and general over-indulgence, I'm usually feeling fat, full, and ready for bed by 9.00 p.m. And I've always found New Year's Eve, or Hogmanay, as we call it in Scotland, to be massively overrated. It's a night that's expected to be bigger and better than any other simply because it's the last in the calendar. Life's best nights are rarely that contrived; you usually stumble into them by accident.

As my year of sobriety draws to a close, I'm continually being asked if I'm raring to have a drink at midnight on New Year's Eve. I was still knocking back tequila at 5.00 a.m. last year, so technically I won't be allowed my first drink until well into New Year's Day. But the thought of a glass of wine or a beer doesn't consume my every waking moment — it's deciding if and when I'll have another drink that does. After 1 January, I'll be free from my pledge, and pondering what I'll do with that freedom is a glimpse into the great unknown. Whatever happens, I'm proud that I've got this far.

On Christmas Eve, the plan is for Loretta to pick me up at 7.00 a.m., and we'll start our nine-hour drive north, to Sydney. At 5.10 a.m., my phone beeps. I wake with a jolt. My first thought is that she must be running late. I fumble in the dark, grumpy at being woken so early. But it's not Loretta. It's Fiona's husband, David, in Edinburgh. He never texts me — something's not right. I squint at the glare on the screen. The message makes no sense. 'Our beautiful son Jude passed away suddenly this afternoon …' Is this is a sick joke? Am I still asleep? I stumble out of bed, hurtling towards the wall, fingers splayed as they scramble for the light switch. Reading the words again, I drop to my knees. The phone bounces on the carpet and the world, changed beyond all recognition, shudders to a stop. My heart thumps so loudly it feels as if the walls are shaking. I wail one word over and over: no.

Fiona and David's Jude, a boy so beautiful he could make godless heathens believe in heavenly creatures, is gone. He was five. How could this have happened? Just over a week ago, he was racing around their home as I chatted to Fiona on Skype. Every now and then, I'd see a flash of blonde hair and hear his cheeky laugh as he dashed past with his big sister, Isla. When he stopped to wave at me, my heart skipped, and I was struck, as I always was, by what a perfect wee soul Fiona and David had created.

I cancel my Sydney trip and spend the rest of the day on the phone to Scotland, trying to piece together what happened. My parents, who have loved Fiona like a daughter since we were kids, are heartbroken. Dad, who got David's message as a text-to-speech voicemail on his answering machine, is distraught. I call Lisa, Jude's godmother, whose three girls are like sisters to Isla and Jude. They're shattered. We cry together as she tells me how it came to this. In the week leading up to Christmas, everything seemed normal: Jude had been playing with Isla and getting excited about Santa coming. But he started to get ill as the week went on; Fiona and David thought he had a chest infection. Three days before Christmas — only two days ago — he started to have problems breathing. His fingers began to turn blue. They took him to hospital, and it quickly became apparent from the looks on the faces of the doctors and nurses that this was more serious than Fiona and David could ever have imagined. There was little time to prepare; Jude died the next day. As I try to process it, I realise that the text message from David came just hours after their boy passed away.

There was nothing the medical team could do — Jude had a large hole in his heart. The doctors said this kind of pulmonary hypertension is a congenital time bomb: it's rare and incurable, and very difficult to diagnose. Even if he had survived, he would have needed a heart–lung transplant. It might have bought him two years, maybe three, at best. He seemed like such a robust boy, who'd never shown any signs of ill health, and yet he was a desperately sick child. It was nothing short of miraculous that he'd survived this long.

As the day goes on, disbelief and desolation come in brutalising waves, like aftershocks in the trail of an earthquake. It feels as if a part of me has been hollowed out; my heart aches for Fiona's loss. She's not able to talk on the phone, but we text, our usual banter replaced by previously unthinkable sentences. I call her mum and tell her how sorry I am. Fiona's her only child. Those grandchildren are everything to her. Her grief is raw and jagged; just hearing her voice cuts me in two. I've never felt more impotent. The phone call leaves me on the floor in howling tears.

Friends come round to offer support, and suggest that if I want a drink, I shouldn't feel bad for having one. It hadn't even crossed my mind. To think that until this morning my biggest worry was whether or not to have a glass of wine is more ridiculous than I can fathom. Even if nobody would blame me for seeking solace in a bottle, it's the last thing I want to do. It's hard enough to cope with this sober. If I get drunk, it might numb the pain for a few hours, but the grief will be more than I can manage tomorrow. Besides, I don't want to block out my emotions, excruciating as they are. Somehow, the pain makes me feel closer to Fiona.

Christmas Day is far from how I imagined it. I spend it with David's brother Mark and his wife, Heather, at their home in Melbourne's bayside suburbs. They're in shock; they can't believe their nephew is gone. Their girls, aged three and 16 months, are too young to understand they've lost a much-loved cousin, but being with them is comforting as we share the loss, clinging to each other for steadiness.

Before I arrived at their place, Fiona texted me to say that she's glad we're all together and she hopes we have a good day with lots of laughter — even in the depths of her grief she's thinking of us. I promise that's what we'll try to do. I dance with the girls, play games, and laugh with them. Over lunch, we smile as we remember Jude for the cheeky little cuddle-monster he was. But when the girls are in bed, the three of us fall apart. We think of Fiona and David waking up on Christmas morning to this foreign world without Jude, his presents wrapped and ready for him to open under a tree he helped to decorate. We think of his partner in crime, his seven-year-old sister, Isla, who asked Fiona if this means she's now an only child.

Mark and I look at flights home, but we can't book until we find out when the funeral will be. The Christmas and New Year holidays mean that all of the arrangements are delayed. If we leave now and find out the funeral's a fortnight away, we risk having to come back to Melbourne for work before it's been held. Waiting is torturous. Every part of me yearns to be back in Scotland.

IT'S NEW YEAR'S Eve: the last day of the most extraordinary year of my life. I'm still in Melbourne; we leave for Scotland in a couple of days. I've been invited to a friend's barbecue to take in the festivities. I don't feel like celebrating, but I'll go. Part of me wants to throw my hands in the air, bemoan the futility of our daily rituals, and retreat into grief. The other part knows I have to live.

As I drive from my flat to the party, it's a stifling hot New Year's Eve night, just as it was this time last year. The drive takes me past my local McDonald's, where, 364 days ago, as I battled with a hangover that felt as if it might kill me, I nearly lost my mind. My heart races a little as I pass it, and I remember how awful I felt that day. And the next day. What a monumental waste of time that now seems, to spend so much of life hung-over, sleeping away my weekends and cowering under the covers, scared of life. I used to tell myself that the places I was going to visit, the friends I cancelled on, or the family I was meaning to call could wait until tomorrow. How cavalier of me to presume those opportunities would always be there.

At the barbecue, people are supportive and offer their condolences. Talking about Jude helps. Although it's all I can think of, I'm reluctant to dwell on it, conscious that this stuff makes some people uncomfortable, and that it is meant to be a party. But Mari-Claire is amazing. She listens for a long time, asks questions about Jude, looks at photos of him, and doesn't flinch when I cry. It turns out that she's going through her own grief — a good friend of hers is in the end stages of terminal cancer. We talk about our sorrow, the kind that can overwhelm us in the most unexpected moments. And we talk about how, in these moments, there is still reason to be thankful: they remind us how lucky we are. For the first time in a week, I feel hopeful.

As midnight approaches and I sip my third ginger beer, my heart is a knot of conflicting emotions. It is, of course, not how I pictured this moment, but there's a sense of achievement at having reached the end of the year without alcohol. There were tough times and countless temptations. I outlasted them all. Yet it's hard to feel proud of a milestone that seems so insignificant compared to the challenge my friend and her husband will face for the rest of their lives. But I know that they will survive this. Fiona is one of the strongest people I know. She's making herself get out of bed; she's continuing to breathe. She's carrying on, for her daughter, for her husband, for herself, and for her darling son, who lived a life filled with love. But for them, like so many of us touched by Jude's death, nothing is the same. No longer can we say this sort of stuff happens to other people. It has revealed that the ground beneath us is shaky; it has underscored our impermanence and made visible the ticking clocks above the heads of those we hold dear. Jude's legacy will be what we do with that knowledge: we will love more fiercely; we will make brave choices, even when we're scared; we will not let our dreams wait until tomorrow.

The countdown begins as we're in the backyard, listening to Lionel Richie's 'All Night Long' turned up loud. I've never felt less like dancing in my life, all night long or otherwise, but I go through the motions. When 2012 arrives, I hug and kiss my friends, and wish them well for the year ahead. Traditionally this day, more than any other, signifies the closing of old chapters and the promise of new beginnings. It's the time when we vow that this year we will be better. My list of new year's resolutions is short — there is only one. It is a reminder and a promise: life's too short to be wasted.

After

MELBOURNE IS UNWELL. On the first day of 2012, the city is teeming with casualties from end-of-year celebrations. I go for a lunchtime walk in the sunshine and see vampires everywhere. They're pale and anguished, recoiling from the light. It feels good to be looking the day in the eye, not hiding in the shadows.

Chris Raine calls to congratulate me on my year without alcohol. We reflect on how much has changed since we first met. *Hello Sunday Morning* has grown from a small network of his friends and acquaintances to a movement of almost 3500 people in Australia, New Zealand, and the United Kingdom. He's been selected as Queensland's nominee for Young Australian of the Year, and I'm so proud of him — he's come a long way from the sober freak at the party in a gimp mask and red undies. For me, it's been the most rewarding, productive year of my life. I feel as if I've achieved more in the last 12 months than I have in the last decade. I learned to run, I sang in public, I saved thousands of dollars, I shed my self-consciousness and danced on a bar with my mother, I took the leap and started grown-up dating, and my dream of writing a book came true. All I had to do was lay off the booze.

Today, as countless Australians wake up to a world of pain, some are drawing a line in the sand. The *Hello Sunday Morning* website has gone into overdrive: one person is signing up every four minutes. It seems there's an appetite for change. Sometimes, I don't think Chris realises just how powerful this thing he started is, but others do. If he can win this award, it will change everything. The publicity would catapult *Hello Sunday Morning* to a new level of community awareness. I can picture a time when taking a break from drinking won't be a big deal. You won't have to cop flak from your mates, convince people you're not a religious zealot, or face claims of being unpatriotic. 'I'm doing *HSM*' will become such an accepted part of the Australian vernacular that it's all you'll need to say.

I'm optimistic, but the shift might take a long time. Economic forecasts predict that Australia's spending on booze will increase by 15 per cent, to reach an annual splurge of more than $29 billion in 2016–17. Consumption is set to rise to more than 11 litres per person — that's about a 4 per cent increase on current drinking rates. It's not suggestive of a nation looking to ease up on its boozing habits. More people will drink at home, with takeaway grog from bottle shops, pubs, and hotels set to account for 80 per cent of spending on booze by 2016. And the more readily available it is, the more we'll drink. Soon, you might not even have to go to a bottle shop: you could pick up a slab in your local 7-Eleven store, or grab a bottle of wine while you're filling your car up at the servo. The Australasian Association of Convenience Stores, representing chains including 7-Eleven, BP, and Caltex Star Mart, has asked the federal productivity commission to consider allowing them to sell booze. In its submission to an inquiry into the retail industry, the group claims that they need to be able to sell booze to counter increasing competition from the two supermarket giants. They argue that a ban on liquor in convenience stores is restricting the Australian convenience industry from a 'potentially crucial revenue stream'.

There's no doubt that this stream is overflowing. The

supermarkets already use booze as a way to entice us into buying groceries or petrol from their chains. Liquorland, owned by Coles, has offered 20 cents off a litre of petrol when buying selected alcohol products. Woolworths knocked 30 cents off a litre for motorists who bought two slabs of beer or pre-mixed spirits instead of one. If the convenience stores are successful, it will mean an extra 4500 outlets across Australia where you can buy booze. Only a wowser would see that as a bad thing, right? But at a time when alcohol-related problems such as domestic violence and sexual assault, known to be linked to bottle-shop density, are on the rise, public-health groups say that adding more places to buy grog would be disastrous.

How do groups such as *Hello Sunday Morning* convey the message that life can be fun without alcohol when it's everywhere we look, even next to the bread and milk? It's tough to convince Aussies to take a break from drinking when alcohol is so ubiquitous — used to commemorate our fallen diggers, back up our sporting heroes, and sell us the notion that it can help us to make friends and find love. As rewarding as my year without booze has been, swimming against the tide has been bloody hard, and at times exhausting. It could be even harder for the next generation of drinkers. As long as laying off the booze leads to claims that you're a boring, un-Australian loser in an environment set up to convince you alcohol makes you cool and socially functional, young people will continue to get pissed for confidence, comfort, and belonging.

Chris is undaunted by the challenge. He thinks that the culture can change, and his goal is 10,000 *HSM* sign-ups by the end of 2012. He's more than a third of the way there already. It's remarkable to think it all started with one guy discovering that confidence, identity, and happiness can't be measured in standard drinks. That idea spread to five of his friends; ten of their friends followed suit. He believes if 10,000 people could find out first-hand that life doesn't have to revolve around booze, the ripple effect might spread far enough to change the nation's drinking culture forever. When that happens, how long before we can truly say that you don't need alcohol to be Australian?

Shortly before I'm due to fly back to Scotland, I receive a letter which addresses that question. It's from the Department of Immigration and Citizenship. After a year spent doing something I was told was distinctly un-Australian, I've become an Australian citizen. The irony makes me laugh. The final legal step is making a pledge of commitment, and I'm invited to do that at a ceremony on 26 January: Australia Day. In the midst of all that's happened, it takes me by surprise. I'm not sure how I feel about it. I've bought a home here. I've been a permanent resident for four years, and lived here for ten, so this is the logical next step. And yet I'm torn. When I applied for citizenship, it wasn't a hugely symbolic gesture; it was mostly so I could vote. Now, it feels as if I'm turning my back on my roots at a time when the need to be Scottish has never been greater. I'm already so far away from Fiona when she needs me, and I worry that by becoming Australian I'll somehow be even more distant. But then my thoughts clear, and I realise that I'll always be Scottish. After this ceremony, I'll just be Australian, too. What my mum calls my 'bigamous love affair' with two countries will continue.

I wonder if the immigration department knows that I haven't had a beer for more than a year. Will I really be 'one of youse' without a drink in my hand? After all, this is the country that brought us 'drinkwear' — in the course of my research, I discovered a Queensland-based company that makes a range of shorts, hats, and T-shirts for the 'drinking enthusiast', with built-in twist-top bottle openers and detachable velcro stubby coolers. The animated advert on their website depicts a bunch of blokes at a barbecue and warns, 'If you're hanging for a cold one, beware the beer lover who hasn't got essential drinkwear, because an Aussie desperate for a beer will try almost anything.' The cartoon characters then injure themselves attempting to open stubbies with various parts of their anatomy. It seems drinking is such an intrinsic part of being Australian, there's a market for clothes that eliminate those crucial lost seconds spent in trying to find a bottle opener; with these garments, you're ready to drink at the drop of a hat. Literally.

Perhaps I won't be issued with a passport until I'm back on the piss. A friend tells me that after I'm sworn in, we'll sing the national anthem and my local mayor will hand me a six-pack of VB as an official welcome to the country. I think he's joking, but I can't be sure. I'll find out in a couple of weeks.

MY TIME IN Edinburgh is gruelling. These homecomings are usually such happy occasions, but this time, nothing is as it should be. The death of a child upends our understanding of the way the universe should operate. It's as if gravity has been suspended; waterfalls are flowing in reverse. Impossible is our new reality.

Normally I can't get to Fiona's house fast enough. Today, I sit in the car outside and wonder how I will put one foot in front of the other. She greets me at the door, and, as we embrace, I am swimming in her grief. I want to fall inside her, absorbing her pain and making it mine. But there's no willing this loss away. Inside their home, Jude's absence feels bigger than the house itself. I'm amazed at how strong she and David are. It's plain that a piece of them is missing, and that they're surviving moment to moment, but there's a calm acceptance of what's happened. They're taking comfort in the five happy years they had with Jude. He was in no distress. Even at the end, he felt no pain.

Fiona says that she stopped saying 'why us?' very early on. She knows it was a medical problem, and that nothing could have saved him. There's no anger or denial, just missing him. Missing him so much it feels like she can't breathe. Lisa's here too, and although none of us — three pals since primary school — could ever have imagined this day, we are together, and there's comfort in that. We drink a lot of tea. We talk and remember, and listen. Fiona tells us about what happened. She knew that it was serious when she saw the number of consultants and doctors streaming in to see Jude in the emergency department. The day after he was admitted, he had an echocardiogram, to provide images of his heart. Nurses were whispering about ventilators. The mood was bleak. Fiona sat with Jude, telling the story of King Arthur and the Knights of the Round Table while he ate Rice Krispies. She knew he wouldn't be home in time for Christmas, but they talked about whether he could see Santa from his hospital window. As she cuddled next to him in bed, a nurse overheard him say that he had the best mummy in the world. What a lovely thing to say, the nurse commented. She wasn't to know that this was a daily occurrence in their house; they were an inseparable duo.

At lunchtime, the cardiologist told them she had some very bad news. A few hours later, Jude slipped out of consciousness. He died in Fiona's arms at 3.10 in the afternoon on Friday 23 December 2011, five years and four months, to the day, after she brought him into the world. Hearing Fiona relive this, it feels as though I might be crushed under the weight of her loss. But she has no tears today. So this is how I need to be for her. I listen, and somehow find a way to hold it together as she tells me how, after Jude was gone, they held him, then washed him and dressed him in clean pyjamas. They said their goodbyes and carried him to the hospital's Chapel of Rest, and laid him in a bed full of teddy bears.

Fiona tells us that she finds herself saying 'at least' a lot. There was a time, just two weeks ago, when there was no room for the notion that there could be something worse than her son being dead. Now, these thoughts sustain her: at least he didn't suffer, at least there's no-one to blame, and at least they still have Isla. At least they were blessed with a boy who enriched their lives every day he was with them.

The impact that Jude's passing has had is clear by the number of mourners who turn up to honour him as he is laid to rest. Five hundred of them, packed into the cathedral where Jude was baptised, and where Lisa and I stood next to Fiona as bridesmaids. The details are too painful. The funeral of a child will always be an unbearably sad occasion — but sadness and tears are not what defined Jude's short life; his was a world filled with laughter and fun. He knew he was loved, and gave love in abundance in return. Even now he's gone, he's still giving love.

Over the eight days I spend at home, there is sadness so intense it sometimes feels as if it will devour me. But there are also moments that raise me up: watching Fiona go through this is more painful than I can bear, but in a strange way I have never loved her more. The strength that she and David have shown as they try to return their daughter's life to some semblance of normality is humbling, and testament to their devotion as parents. My love for Lisa, her heart broken by the loss of her godson and her family's grief, has been magnified by her loyal and gentle attention to Fiona and her family in their darkest hours. Of course we'd all give anything to have Jude back, but this deeper, richly textured love he has fostered among us is something special. It is his gift to us.

The day after the funeral, I catch up with a bunch of old school friends for a pub lunch. Some of them I know well, while some of them I haven't seen since the day we left high school. We gather because we feel helpless. Being together feels like we're doing something. So much time has passed since we last met, but there's no awkwardness, only affection, sympathy, and a common bond of history. When we were 20 and one of our high-school classmates died suddenly, most of us went to the funeral and piled into our local afterwards. We got hammered, singing and crying, and telling cracking tales about the friend we'd lost. The wake went on well into the night. In Scotland, farewelling the dead with a big drinking session is all part of the grieving process.

My year without alcohol is officially over; I could have a drink if I want to. But when we meet, I don't want booze. I've brought a bag of old photographs, and we look at ourselves on school trips and at teenage parties and twenty-firsts, so young and carefree. We laugh at our clothes, our hairstyles, and the boyfriends and girlfriends we swore we couldn't live without, but whose faces have faded from memory. Fiona and I are together in so many pictures, looking dorky, hugging and dancing and getting drunk, celebrating our wins and toasting our youth. In one picture, we must be about 22. Our arms are intertwined and our bodies so close we look like Siamese twins. I touch the photograph, looking into the eyes of this girl, who is often mistaken for my sister. My darling Fee. How I wish I could save her from what lies ahead.

After we leave the pub, five of us take a walk along Portobello beach promenade. It's a chilly Sunday afternoon, with a bracing wind. The sun is setting, turning the horizon into a beautiful fleece of amber and pink. We walk towards it, huddled together. It's clear from the conversation how moving this loss has been for all of us, even for those who never met Jude. How could this happen? It's not right. None of this is right. As we walk, we talk about the things that have been consuming my mind: how it's shocked us into paying greater respect to what we have, where we came from, and where we want to be. I don't know them as I once did, and we may not talk for another ten years, but right now I feel a profound sense of closeness to these old school friends. The ties of our shared past are now interwoven with these bonds of grief and renewed perspective. I'm glad that I haven't had a drink today. I want to experience these feelings in all their depth — life is so much richer when you let yourself feel. When we say goodbye, there's an intensity to the hugs that buoys me. Jude's life means something. Somehow this tragedy has lifted us up. We are better people for it.

BACK IN MELBOURNE, I try to return to something akin to normal. The first week is tough. On Friday night, after a particularly bad day at work, I catch up with Kath and Loretta for dinner at a bar near my place. I don't feel like it at all. When I arrive, I tell them that I'm really flat and won't stay long because I just want to hibernate. They convince me to stay and talk. They know how much I'm struggling. Both of them have spent time with Fiona: Kath met her when we went to Scotland last year, and we all danced till the wee small hours; Loretta had an afternoon of sampling malt whiskies with Fiona and Mum a few years ago, during a visit to Edinburgh.

I decide not to leave, and we end up having a wonderful night together. I stick to water while they have wine, but I don't feel as if I'm missing out. We talk about our plans for the future, our hopes, and our fears. We vow to always be daring, and not sit passively by as life wanders past. It's as if, being with them, I've been plugged in — I can feel myself recharging. As they build me up, I have one of those sweet moments of clarity where I can see how blessed I am to have these two beautiful women in my world. At a time when I'm trying to process my grief, their friendship is life-affirming. I'm reflecting on this on the tram ride to work the next day; I text them both to say how much their friendship means to me. The perspective Jude's passing has brought is allowing me to feel things I've never felt. It's helped me see what's right there in front of me.

Staying true to my *carpe diem* pledge, I decide to say yes to something that scares me. A friend, Jo, is getting married in a few weeks. She heard about my music-school gig and has asked me to be one of the singers in a wedding band with some of the couple's friends. Initially I thought, I can't do it; I've got too much work to do. Loretta and Kath made me see that this was an excuse. The thought of singing in front of 100 wedding guests petrifies me, but I've discovered that most of the things worth doing in life are scary — it's what makes the rewards that much greater.

I turn up to my first rehearsal in a real studio, with a bunch of musicians who are so talented, it's intimidating just to stand next to them. It's a hot, sticky night, and everyone's cooling down with a beer or a glass of wine. With all that's happened these last few weeks, I've shelved thoughts of when I might drink again. Tonight, I stay on water, but it brings my mind back to the decision ahead of me. I wonder if, where, and when I should have my first drink. My worries about what will happen when I invite alcohol back into my life are less pronounced than they were a few weeks ago. Part of me is still nervous that Jon Currie's elastic-band analogy will prove prophetic and that my drinking habits will quickly snap back to old ways, but the part of me that's just had the cruellest of life lessons believes I won't allow that to happen.

When it's my turn to step up to the mike in the studio, I rock out. The buzz is electrifying, and it's such a stress relief. By the end of the night I feel as if I've run a half-marathon; the tension has gone from my body. It is more fun than I've had in a very long time.

ON THE MORNING of my citizenship ceremony, I'm quite excited. It feels like a big occasion, a festival of me, like my graduation or my 21st birthday. But hopefully this time I'll remember all of it tomorrow. I dress appropriately, in a green dress with a gold cardigan and handbag. Whether I'm drinking or not, no-one can accuse me of being un-Australian in these colours.

Reading *The Age* as I get ready, I see a story that puts the day in context. New figures have revealed that Australia Day is the number-one holiday for heavy drinking, assaults, and car accidents among young people. On this day, more under-25s drink too much, ending up in hospital in higher numbers than on any other public holiday. There are more than double the usual number of ambulance callouts, and a 50 per cent increase in emergency-department presentations. Injuries for assaults also double on Australia Day.

Somewhere along the way, young people have learned that to be
a true-blue Aussie, you need to get plastered. I'm not sure it's always
been like this. I've only been here ten years, but it seems as if the link
between alcoholic obliteration and national pride has become more
pronounced in the last few years. I'm usually working on Australia
Day, so this is one holiday with which I don't have a drunken history,
but last year I remember leaving work about 6.00 p.m., and seeing
hoards of teenagers and 20-somethings pouring out of a tram coming
from St Kilda Beach. Draped in Aussie flags, and wearing bikinis,
hats, and tattoos of the flag, many of them were blind drunk. The
mood didn't seem celebratory. I'm not sure if any of them could have
articulated what it was their boozing was commemorating.

Our national leaders don't always help. At the Australia-versus-
India test match at the Sydney Cricket Ground earlier this month,
former prime minister Bob Hawke made a hero of himself, not for
the first time, by sculling a beer. As he walked through the crowd,
he was handed a cold one, with a supporter yelling out, 'One for
the country, Robert.' With a backdrop of shirtless men cheering
and playing bongo drums, 82-year-old Hawkie knocked back the
entire beer in one long gulp, to the delight of the crowd. Even the
police officers laughed. His sculling was a sign of his patriotism,
with one supporter explaining, 'He's just a great Aussie bloke.' Prime
Minister Julia Gillard would later remark that Hawke got more
media attention for downing that beer than she did for announcing
$95 million in cricket funding, musing that next time she made an
announcement she should do it with a beer in her hand.

Sadly, Chris misses out on Young Australian of the Year. He was
among a field of talented high achievers, but it's disappointing not to
see him get the recognition he deserves. A week later, *Hello Sunday
Morning* is knocked back for a community grant under the federal
government's National Binge Drinking Strategy. Politicians talk a
good game about wanting to change the culture around alcohol, but

when faced with someone who has a proven method of doing that, they look the other way.

As I drive to Coburg Town Hall for my citizenship ceremony, it's a beautiful morning. There's a laid-back holiday feel to the streets, which are quieter than usual, and it does seem that most of Melbourne is already in the party mood. A guy riding a bike one-handed is swigging a Corona. Another bloke walking across the street alone is drinking a Boag's. A couple struggle with a slab and an esky as they head to the tram stop. It's as if being caught in public without alcohol on this day is unpatriotic. By the time I arrive at the town hall and mingle with my fellow citizens-to-be, I've already decided that today is not the day I'll have my first drink. One thing I've learned from a year of abstinence is that drinking just for the sake of it is pointless. Having a beer simply because it's Australia Day seems a poor reason to start drinking, especially when I don't even feel like alcohol.

Fifteen friends turn up to watch me take the pledge. I feel very much loved. There are numerous speeches from various local, state, and federal politicians. In his address, the mayor of Moreland City Council tells us that no-one expects we will forget our families or our homeland. 'This makes you the person that you are,' he says. 'These experiences will remain treasured memories. Leaving your home country means moving from the known to the unknown.' After the month I've just experienced, I couldn't agree more.

Finally, the time comes to make our pledge. Eighty of us stand and together recite the words, 'From this time forward, I pledge my loyalty to Australia and its people, whose democratic beliefs I share, whose rights and liberties I respect, and whose laws I will uphold and obey.' The room erupts in applause, my little corner of fans leading the charge. The mayor then asks us to repeat one sentence: 'I am Australian.' As I say the words, I'm more emotional than I expected. I feel proud to be part of this great nation. I look at my friends, cheering me on as they welcome me officially into the fold. I'm happy to be an Australian if being Australian means that I belong to them. Yet that familiar heart-torn feeling lingers. I think of the ones I love in Scotland: I think of Fiona, of Mum and Dad and Lisa. I'm theirs too. I hope I always will be.

When my name's called, I walk up to the mayor and wait to see what he gives me. There's no six-pack of beer. Instead, I receive a native sapling and a certificate. My entourage goes wild. Blinking against a lightning storm of cameras flashing, the mayor quips that I have more paparazzi than Elle Macpherson.

Later, in a beer garden, my friends propose a toast to me, their new Australian. I raise my lemonade to their beer. Afterwards, we go to another friend's house for a barbecue. There are more congratulations and hugs at my newfound Aussieness. It's a glorious afternoon. It strikes me that this is the essence of being Australian: spending time with family and friends on a summer's day at a backyard barbecue. I don't need a drink in my hand to feel part of that. Having a beer is something you enjoy. It's not who you are. It's not where you came from. Whether I'm Australian or Scottish, my identity is no longer tied to alcohol.

IT FEELS LIKE the right time. I'm at Jo and Jamie's wedding. I've just watched them get married in a beautiful garden ceremony on a perfect Saturday afternoon in a country town north-west of Melbourne. Walking to the reception with friends, I decide that it would be nice to have a drink to toast this happy occasion. It's been nearly 14 months since my last; I've smashed the challenge. What am I waiting for? If I want to know if I can drink without alcohol controlling me, what better test than a weekend away at a wedding, with a free bar that's open till 3.00 a.m.

At the venue, my friend Megan goes to the bar to buy champagne and spreads word that I'm about to have my first drink. I'm told to wait a few minutes while more friends queue at the bar for their own drinks to toast me with. I've waited 413 days — nearly 14 months. A few more minutes won't hurt. Some people start filming, as if they're about to witness a dog walking on its hind legs. What's going to happen? Will I collapse in a drunken heap the moment that first drop of alcohol is absorbed into my bloodstream? Perhaps I'll vomit, or break out in a rash. My biggest worry is where I'll be at the end of the night. Will I morph into a shambolic Shane MacGowan/Keith Richards–inspired inebriate who jumps on the table, downs a bottle of Scotch, and performs a striptease?

Megan comes back and puts the glass of champagne in front of me. It fizzes like a cartoon bomb. I stare at it, biting my lip. My hands are clammy. Loretta, sitting on a stool next to me, puts an arm around my waist and gives me a squeeze. 'It's all good.'

I'm not so sure. After this long without a drink, I have no idea where this glass of champers will take me. A friend said recently that it was like I'd been re-virginated. As if I'm waiting for my first time, scared it will hurt or that I'll make a fool of myself.

The other girls come back from the bar, and I raise my glass to theirs. There is whooping and cheering and flashing cameras. It's lovely that everyone wants to be part of this momentous occasion, but I'm not sure if they're cheering my achievement or the fact I've finally seen the light. I feel like an exiled cult member welcomed back into the sect, after realising that life on the outside was just as unfulfilling as I'd been warned.

As I reach over to clink glasses with those on the other side of the table, my champagne flute is snatched away by a mischievous friend. He's shouting, 'Don't do it,' to jeers. Part of me wonders if maybe I should just let him keep it.

He hands it back and I raise the glass to my lips. I take a sip and wait.

'How do you feel?' I'm asked before I've set the glass down on the table. Everyone's staring and grinning.

'I don't know,' I say. 'It's hard to explain.' But honestly, it feels like a massive anticlimax. There's no rush of energy like there was when I inadvertently had a hit of booze at the cocktail party — I'm not buzzing, or consumed by thoughts of getting drunk. Yet this night has a long way to go. 'Ask me again in three hours, when I'm slumped in a corner,' I joke. If old habits are ever going to come back, then this night, with a stage on which I'll soon be performing and a dance floor filled with good friends, would be the occasion.

I drink my bubbly very slowly, worried that it will go straight to my head and leave me incapable of singing. An hour passes and I'm still only halfway through. Then I realise I'm not actually that keen on champagne. Why am I drinking this? I leave the half-filled glass on a table, proud of myself for walking away from alcohol I'm not enjoying — something I've rarely done before. What I really want is a beer. Someone gets me a pot of my favourite pale ale. I look at the frothy head, inhaling its rich aroma before bringing it to my lips. This is something I've really missed.

When I take a sip, I'm disappointed. It tastes ordinary. Another hour passes, and the half-pot of beer I have left has turned flat and warm. I stop drinking it. I thought that after nearly 14 months without booze, half a glass of champers and half a beer would be enough to leave me reeling. Or at least give me a buzz. But I feel no effects.

This turns out to be a good thing. When it's my turn to get on stage with the wedding band, to belt out the rock classic 'What I Like About You', I'm completely lucid. The dance floor fills up, friends cheer, and I'm on a natural high. In another song, the band drops out, leaving me singing a verse *a cappella* to a hushed audience. It should be scary, but it's not. In fact, the experience is so exhilarating that I can feel the hairs on the back of my arms standing up. Gripping the microphone, my eyes half closed under the lights, I think of my 413 days without alcohol. And I think of Jude's short life. The two things that have forever changed my view of the world. They brought me here, to this stage. I'm no longer the scared procrastinator, cowering under the covers with my dreams still inside me. I hope I never will be again.

Our finale, in which we form a supergroup with the other wedding band and perform the Rolling Stones' classic 'Jumpin' Jack Flash', nearly brings the house down. Watching her friends sing for her, the bride is moved to tears. Being involved in this band on such a happy occasion is one of the most fulfilling experiences I've ever had. If this wedding had taken place a year ago, I'd probably have got hammered first to give me courage. What a waste it would have been if I couldn't remember the performance the next day.

I have another beer after the set, but again it goes flat and warm as I struggle to drink it. It just tastes bad. I feel gassy and bloated. All I want to do is drink water. A friend tells me to persevere: if I want to get my drinking boots back, I'm going to have to put in the hard yards. I feel like I'm 13 and trying to push through the foul taste of alcohol to get the desired result. The difference this time is that I don't really want to get drunk. My friends are hitting it hard and having a great time, but after two half-finished pots of beer over four hours, I already taste the hangover. And I'm hit by a wave of melancholy that I can't quite explain. Maybe the alcohol is having a depressive effect — I've hardly drunk anything, but the effect on my nervous system is probably amplified after so long without it. Part of the sadness also comes, I think, from knowing that this is the end of a chapter. The challenge is over, and now I'm just like everyone else. How many times did I feel on the outside of the group this last year? Yet now that I'm back inside it, I'm already missing my difference.

I put the beer down and start drinking water. It doesn't stop me from dancing. It's the complete opposite of how I expected this night would end up when I decided to have a drink. I worried that alcohol would have such a hold on me, I'd lose control at the first taste. Part of me is thrilled to realise that maybe I can be one of those people who drinks moderately. The other part thinks, settle down, there's a long way to go.

I don't have another drink for the rest of the night. I decide that walking a kilometre up a steep hill in stilettos and waking up with a hangover that leaves me despondent is too big a price to pay for being drunk. I leave the wedding at 2.00 a.m., sober and driving, as I'd originally planned. I go to sleep wondering if maybe I've cracked it. Everything in moderation. Dad would be so proud.

A FEW DAYS later, I catch up with Kath for dinner, and something changes. I have my first glass of wine in nearly 14 months. It tastes great. The next one tastes even better. That buzz is back. I go home after two glasses, but I know that if Kath wasn't driving and didn't have to leave early, I'd have ordered another, and maybe another after that. I've no desire to buy a bottle on the way home and drink on my own, but I do sense that my transition to moderate drinking isn't going to be as smooth as I thought.

Tonight, the indifference I felt towards drinking at the wedding is replaced by feelings of excitement. After so long without it, I'd forgotten how enjoyable that tipsy feeling can be. It doesn't necessarily mean I'm on a fast track to annihilation, but it makes me cautious. Can I stop at that fun, tipsy stage, or will I always crave more?

It reminds me of an article that my editor emailed me a few weeks ago, helpfully pointing out how booze makes us happy. Researchers from the University of California managed to pinpoint the exact regions in the brain that are excited by alcohol. Previously, studies on animals had shown that drinking creates a pleasurable effect by releasing endorphins, the feel-good chemicals, in the brain, but this study was the first to prove the effect in humans. The researchers examined the brains of heavy drinkers and compared them to moderate drinkers. The more endorphins that were released, the more pleasure all participants felt. What was fascinating was that as endorphin levels increased, the heavy drinkers felt more pleasure than those in the control group. This suggests, the scientists said, that the brains of heavy drinkers are altered in some way to make them more likely to find alcohol enjoyable. The greater the feelings of pleasure, the more they drink. Even when it's 3.00 a.m., they're on their 12th beer, and they've just thrown up in a post-box.

Jon Currie warned me that although my brain scan showed no structural damage, the neuropsychological tests and my drinking history suggest that I may have difficulty avoiding those big binges. Perhaps my brain's pleasure centre is more susceptible to alcohol's effects than the average drinker. I think of Will and his 18 cans a day, and wonder if maybe I *am* destined for the 'High Sobriety' club. I thought that we were so different because I drank less than him. But after a year without booze, addiction is not as black-and-white as I once thought — there are so many shades of grey. I'm reminded of another comment that a reader left at the end of my confessional *Sunday Age* article. He was a big drinker who loved a party, but it was getting out of hand, so he took a month off the grog. He felt great and thought he could be a moderate drinker. Soon, old habits sneaked up and booze was back in control. He said he was convinced he was the type of alcoholic who can only operate in polar opposites — he can abstain, but only if it is completely. 'The true definition of alcoholic liberty is moderation,' he said.

That's the challenge ahead for me. I don't want to be counting drinks and prostrating myself if I have a big night. But I'd like to feel that if I get drunk it's a choice, not an accident. If it turns out that I can't choose productive Sunday mornings over Saturday nights I don't enjoy and can't remember, or if I can't choose getting things done over feeling done in, maybe I'll have to part company with my old friend booze for good. Whatever happens, I know now that alcohol does not define me. Getting drunk does not make me more Scottish or Australian, nor does it make me a better daughter, friend, aunty, or sister. I don't need a beer in my hand to be accepted as a journalist, a writer, or a footy fan. I stayed sober for more than a year, and I was still all of those things. Without booze, I loved, laughed, and lost. Life did not stop. But it certainly did change.

And then what?

IT'S FRIDAY NIGHT in a busy bar in Melbourne's inner north. There's a buzz in the air — that intoxicating sense of promise and possibility that comes with the first glimpse of the weekend. I'm three beers and one cocktail deep. My eyes dart across the menu, excited by what I might try next. I've never been more enthusiastic about a night of drinking. The options are endless — more than 100 beers, ciders, wines, spirits, cocktails, and pre-mixed drinks. Every single one of them — barring a lone gin and tonic — is alcohol-free.

It's more than a decade since my first year off the booze came to a close, and it's hard to fathom how much things have changed. The fact I'm sinking 'zero' beers at Australia's first permanent non-alcoholic bar is emblematic of a culture that has shifted immeasurably.

At the beginning of this book, you may recall I was offered a free shot of vodka at my local pub to see if I could 'pass the challenge', so alien was the concept of sobriety as a legitimate lifestyle choice or the idea that someone might want to spend time in a bar without drinking alcohol. Now, my local is Brunswick Aces, a thriving alcohol-free watering hole; the 'non-alc' drinks sector is the nation's fastest-growing beverage category; and sobriety is being rebranded in a way that has become, dare I say it, cool.

Welcome to the sober-curious age. It's a term coined by journalist Ruby Warrington, who wrote a bestselling memoir of the same name, tapping into a growing interest in no- or low-alcohol living. It offers a palatable entry point to those who are interested in what life without booze could look like but don't want to be saddled with the stigma of being labelled a sober bore or a problem drinker. Far more socially acceptable to say you're sober-curious than to call yourself a wowser, a raging alcoholic, or a hopeless binge drinker. This clever shift in marketing has helped advance a trend that has slowly been building for years, as a more health-conscious community looks to wean itself off a cultural dependence on drinking. Sobriety is back in fashion, and I'm so here for it.

For my next drink, I opt for a 'Stark Reality' — a martini-inspired cocktail that the bar has named after me, their neighbourhood sober ambassador. I savour the delicate flavours, marvelling at how far we've come. Every table is filled with chattering people actively choosing to spend their Friday night alcohol-free. When Steve Lawrence, one of Brunswick Aces' founders, first outlined his vision for this place at the official launch party, it moved me to tears. He wanted to create a space where people feel like they belong. A place where non-drinkers aren't treated like an afterthought, or sold lesser products in inferior glassware. After so long feeling like a pariah exiled to the social wilderness, walking into a bar where you're openly celebrated for the very thing that once left you on the outer is like finding a long-lost family.

The name of my signature cocktail is fitting. It sums up how I feel three years into my second crack at alcohol-free living. Sobriety is raw, and it's real, and it strips you bare. It allows you to see yourself close-up and in sharp focus. Sometimes the stark reality of that can be confronting, but it also brings a sense of fulfilment and clarity that is so rewarding. It's hard to imagine alcohol ever again occupying the space in my life it once did.

But I'd be lying if I said the road to get here was easy. So much has changed, for my own relationship with alcohol and for the wider drinking culture — which I'll return to later — but let's start with me.

At the end of my initial year off the booze, I went back to drinking — a decision that was an enormous disappointment to many readers who were more invested in my journey than I could ever have anticipated when I embarked on what was always meant to be a year-long personal experiment. Some were downright furious, and they didn't shy away from telling me. Had I learned nothing? How could I have so many revelations about the role of alcohol in my life and then welcome it back like a toxic friend? There was a quiet desperation in some of their questions. 'How do you drink now?' 'Have you been able to master moderation?' It was unsettling to find so many people had tied their relationship with alcohol to mine.

In my defence, I didn't ask to become the poster girl for sobriety — although, alarmingly, this headline was placed above my face on the front page of one of the British broadsheets when the book was released in the UK. The pressure was intense. People approached me in bars, an eyebrow raised towards my glass of wine as they asked, 'Didn't you write a book about sobriety?' I felt like I was failing an entire community who wanted my story to have a neat, redemptive ending that offered hope for their own salvation. Life is rarely that simple. Like so many of the moving cogs that make up the human condition, what happened after my year of sobriety was clunky, complex, and challenging.

Initially, my relationship with alcohol was in balance. There were far more social occasions when I chose not to drink rather than automatically reach for a beer. I was mindful of my reasons for wanting to drink, and consciously opted not to if the underlying driver was anxiety, loneliness, boredom, or a desire to fit in. I felt I'd mastered what one reader described as the 'true definition of alcoholic liberation' — moderation. I carried on as a mindful drinker for a year or so, and really believed this would be my new normal.

But, gradually, old habits crept back in. I wasn't stopping at one or two. The craving for more intensified, and the hangovers returned, precipitated by hazy nights that began with a couple of wines and ended in a fog of regret and broken promises. I didn't see it at the time, but I was using alcohol as an anaesthetic — a quick way to not feel the very big feelings threatening to engulf me.

My return to old drinking ways coincided with a turbulent period in my life that turned everything I knew about myself on its head. When this book was first released, to my great surprise it became a bestseller, and I was propelled into a whirlwind of book tours, TV and radio appearances, and the kind of public adulation I wasn't emotionally equipped to handle. On paper I had it all — my dream job as a campaigning journalist, a bestselling book, great friends and family, and a revolving door of clearly inappropriate but distractingly attractive men. I was living my best life. Until I wasn't. It turns out that getting everything you've ever wanted — only to find that it's not enough because underneath it all you don't believe *you* are enough — is the perfect recipe for an existential meltdown.

Towards the end of 2014, 18 months after realising a childhood dream to become a published author, I experienced a prolonged and debilitating mental health crisis I nearly didn't survive. I'd wrestled with anxiety for most of my life, and had battled through depression as a teenager, but this was unlike anything I'd ever experienced. I felt like I was shattering into a thousand pieces. My psychologist would later rebrand this breakdown as a 'breakthrough', because it's often after these moments that crack us open that we piece ourselves back together with the courage and strength to find out who we really are. This journey, and an exploration of how the relentless pursuit of happiness is making us miserable, is one I documented in my second book, *Happy Never After: why the happiness fairytale is driving us mad (and how I flipped the script)*, so I won't rehash it here (although I would humbly invite you to read it).

During that struggle to rebuild myself, I began, grudgingly, to acknowledge that drinking was incompatible with reclaiming my mental health. In the recovery process, I went for months without drinking, accepting that this was the wisest decision for me at that moment in time. But when I was through the eye of the storm, I always returned to alcohol. It would take five more years, a metric shit ton of therapy, and a series of drunken near-misses before I realised that my break-up with booze probably needed to be a permanent separation.

* * *

I'M OFTEN ASKED to pinpoint the exact moment I knew I couldn't continue drinking. People are keen to hear about my 'rock bottom' — the mortifying incident so catastrophically bad that I had no choice but to change. The notion that we must experience a life-altering disaster before we realise our drinking is a problem is, in itself, problematic. Rock bottom is a cultural trope that conveniently separates those *desperate alcoholics* and *dysfunctional drinkers* from the rest of us who just like to get loose and scull a beer or ten on a Saturday night. It offers comfort to those who want to believe their drinking is fine. I haven't crashed my car, blown up my marriage, or roundhouse-kicked my boss in the head at the office Christmas party, so there's no problem here.

This is my thinking as I return to drinking and find that moderation is more of a challenge than I'd anticipated: *it's not that bad. I only drink socially. I'm not drinking any more than most of my friends. I can slow down, but I don't need to stop.* It's pure denial. I might not have hit rock bottom, but pieces of the cliff face are crumbling in my hands as I cling on for dear life on the descent.

There is the time I get so drunk at a friend's wedding I make out with a stranger and have no recollection of the bride getting up with the band to sing to her new husband. When seeing the video on Instagram the following day, I message a friend to ask him exactly how hammered a person would have to be to not have even the faintest skerrick of a memory of such a significant moment. Only, I don't send these words to him, but inadvertently text them to the CEO of an organisation with whom I'm currently in contract negotiations for a new dream role. Luckily for me, she has a sense of humour.

There's the time I fall on my face leaving a dinner party at a friend's parents' house, peeling my head off the footpath to reveal, to the horrified looks of those around me, a chipped tooth, a deep gash to my nose, and dozens of grazes on my chin. I wake up looking like I've been assaulted. I'm so embarrassed I don't leave the house for two days.

Then there's the midweek knock-off drinks at the pub with workmates at *The Age*, when I hook up with a 24-year-old reporter from *The Daily Mail*, as I loudly proclaim, '*The* Daily Mail *is a cancer*' (that much I stand by) while shoving my hand up the back of his shirt and announcing, '*I may be nearly 40, but fuck yeah, I've still got it!*' The keepsakes from that one-night stand include a broken bed frame, a permanent scar on my knee from falling out of an Uber onto broken glass in the gutter, and three frantic hours the next morning trying to locate the string of a tampon I forgot I was wearing and that had become lodged so deep I nearly had to go to the emergency department to have it removed.

I laugh it all off because I need to believe it's funny. These are battle stories to regale my friends with. Perhaps Starkers the wild party girl is just who I am, and fighting this reality is denying my true nature. I don't want to admit that, after a transformative year off the booze, I've regressed to an unreformed version of myself. So

I find new and inventive ways to justify my debauched behaviour. It's not like every time I drink something bad happens. There are far more uneventful nights than nights of shame. I'm trying desperately to ignore the irrefutable reality that, while fucked-up shit doesn't happen every time I drink, every time I fuck up, I'm drinking.

I'm regularly waking up to a phone that's a crime scene for mistakes. Booty calling mediocre men who have long since lost interest in me. Drunk dialling my best mate 16 times at 3.00 a.m. Frustrated when he doesn't answer, I leave a string of increasingly abusive text messages and voicemails, outlining all the ways in which he's a shit friend who hates me. None of it is based in reality. But those deep emotional issues and worst insecurities that stretch all the way back to childhood — which I'm able to methodically work through in the supported space of therapy — are wildly uncontained when I'm drunk.

Some things I do I can't take back. I hurt people I care about, and break at least one friendship beyond repair. Most of the time, I don't even remember what I've done. Whole chunks of my evening are lost to me. This may be partly due to the antidepressants I'm taking, which really shouldn't be mixed with alcohol. But also, since my sober year, my tolerance is lower, and it doesn't take as much to feel blind drunk. And the older you get, the greater toll alcohol takes. You have less muscle and more fat, meaning you can drink the same as you did when you were younger but you have a higher blood-alcohol concentration, so you get more drunk. It's the perfect storm for memory loss and inebriated indiscretions.

I've conveniently filtered out everything the addiction specialist told me about the significant risk of brain impairment that can come from repeated episodes of blackout drinking. Of course, he also warned that this type of cognitive dissonance — compulsive pleasure-seeking, despite knowing the consequences — is the very definition of 'premalignant addiction'.

There is a part of me — that intuitive, internal voice — trying desperately to alert me to the path my life will take if I don't change direction. I can feel it, niggling away on the periphery of my consciousness. But it's a whisper I'm not ready or able to hear. Alcohol makes so much noise. It screams at me to stop being such a drama queen, that I deserve a drink for all my hard work, that this is perfectly normal behaviour, and everyone else is doing it, so why can't I?

There is no rock bottom. Perhaps if there had been, it would have been harder to ignore my instincts and lie to myself about how things were tracking. As Millie Gooch points out in her book *The Sober Girl Society's Handbook*, if your house was on fire, you wouldn't wait until it burned to the ground before you put out the blaze. The flames are starting to lick at my ankles, but I'm in a stupefied state of paralysis, burning alive in increments. I am the proverbial boiling frog, the heat rising so gradually that I almost don't notice I'm cooked.

It's a particularly raucous party at my apartment in June 2019 that finally forces me to put out the fire. Australia's conservative Coalition government has, quite unexpectedly, been re-elected, and, like many of my liberal-minded friends, I'm depressed by the prospect of another three years of being governed by a party of elitist private school boys who forced the LGBTQIA+ community into a hateful and damaging public vote on their right to marry, and a prime minister so deep in denial about the threat of climate change that he famously embraced a lump of coal during parliamentary question time.

I call it the 'End of the World Party', writing in the Facebook invite: 'It's official: the world is fukt. The planet is cooked and so are the majority of Australians.' I ask my friends to join me to 'party like there's no tomorrow' as we 'numb the pain with a night of unadulterated hedonism'.

And that's exactly what it was. Or so I'm told. I have no recollection of anything from 9.00 p.m. onwards. After sinking several Fireball shots, then proceeding to smoke too much weed, and knocking back half a bottle of wine and some particularly potent vodka jelly shots, I was gone. By all accounts, it was an epic party, but the night comes back to me only in flashes, like grainy, staccato images played on an old projector. Saying something tactless — what and to whom, I don't know. A stumble and the sound of breaking glass. An argument with a faceless human who had hijacked my carefully curated playlist to blast out some tuneless rap that I dramatically declared I simply couldn't bear. A glancing look from my best friend, held a second too long — a wordless moment heavy with disappointment. Quietly weeping in my bedroom because I was so wasted I just wanted people to leave so I could sleep.

The next morning, I wake up to an apartment that looks like a warzone. My stomach lurches as I inhale a putrid mix of musty cigarettes, stale beer stomped into sticky floorboards, and the faint hint of spilled amyl nitrate. I spend two hours on the clean-up, shuffling around like a reanimated corpse, scooping tubs of congealed dip, half-empty bottles, and yellowing wedges of hardened cheese into bin bags, while fighting the urge to hurl. I vacuum the entire apartment, and mop the kitchen and lounge room floors twice, but still the smell lingers. The assault on my senses is an added insult to a body already battered by the night before.

But orders of magnitude worse than my physical discomfort is the crippling hangxiety — that familiar sense of dread and mortification that wraps around me like a hair shirt. In recent times, it has become a common occurrence. My heart and mind race as if I've been mainlining amphetamines. *What did I say? What did I do? Who is waiting for my apology?* I try to pinpoint the root of the feeling, but it has no edges, nothing tangible to grip. Just an amorphous sense of wrongness. An uneasiness so heavy I might suffocate under its weight. Beneath it all, the white-hot burn of shame. I'd been looking forward to this night for so long, and I can't even remember it. Why am I like this? What the fuck is wrong with me?

I lie on the couch under a blanket in the foetal position watching *Fleabag* — vaguely comforted by the neurotic exploits of a woman whose life is also a raging bin fire — and order McDonalds. At least this time there is no panic attack in the car. One of the questionable upsides to the 21st century's advancing technology is the unalienable right to have cheap, highly processed junk food delivered to your door at all hours of the day and night. But as I chew on my sad burger, my mind melting down with hangxiety and regret, I can't deny the parallels to that epic hangover that led to my first year off the booze. How am I back here again?

It's another three weeks before I find the strength to quit drinking. It comes after a series of days I've come to know as 'Suicide Tuesday'. In the immediate aftermath of my big weekends, when the hyper-aroused state of hangxiety has subsided, I often find myself slumping into a depression. It usually hits on a Tuesday and can last days, sometimes weeks. It's the same serotonin-depleted crash in mood I experienced in my early 20s after taking weekend party drugs, and it's the reason I haven't dabbled since. And yet, here I am, two decades later, experiencing the same dizzying fluctuations — this time, precipitated by alcohol. I try to explain the mood changes as nothing more than a natural by-product of a brain predisposed to anxiety, entirely unrelated to drinking. But the inner knowing that is frantically trying to get my attention urges me not to turn away from the truth. Soon, it becomes impossible to ignore. The evidence is there in glorious technicolour.

I keep a mood diary on my phone, using an app called Mood Flow as a factual record of my emotional health. It's a helpful reference point on the days when my mind tricks me into believing everything is always terrible and I've forever been broken. I assign my moods five colours: dark blue is an awful day; light blue is bad; beige is average; pink is good; and hot pink is for those days when the stars feel so perfectly aligned you want to high-five strangers and dance naked in the rain. The run of dark-blue days in the wake of my nights of heavy drinking is unquestionable. What goes up must come down. And when your baseline is a state of utter depletion, the down is a sheer drop to oblivion.

During sessions with my psychologist, Veronica, we often discuss the nauseating rollercoaster ride my drinking is taking me on. I still can't, or won't, make the link. At this point, I've been in therapy for five years, and the work we've done together has been transformative. I have no doubt it saved my life several times over. Veronica is helping me untangle the gnarly roots of my anxiety — a forensic and painstaking excavation of all the hurt from my past. The high school bullying that bred self-loathing and shame, the complicated family issues from childhood that shaped my life choices for decades, and the distorted view these issues gave me of myself and my value. But we've reached a point where I feel stuck. There are more layers, but I can't get deep enough to peel them back.

It's confronting facing the parts of yourself you've been running from for years, the parts you've neglected or denied as a form of self-protection. Sometimes the stark reality of what you uncover in therapy is so unpalatable you can't bear to look. So I don't. Drinking helps me obscure from view the parts I'm not ready to face. But on some level I know that continuing to cloud my vision for fear of what I'll see is not a sustainable or healthy way to live.

At the centre of the work I do with Veronica is a reimagining of my life's meaning. She asks me to reflect on whether the way I'm living leaves me with a sense of expansion. Or does it feel like I'm contracting, becoming a diminished version of myself? She also encourages me to identify the core values by which I want to live — foundation stones to anchor my thoughts, behaviours, and decisions.

I come to see that a full and authentic life can only be lived if it is underpinned by values of integrity, compassion, kindness, and clear-eyed honesty — to those around me and to myself.

On one particularly grim Suicide Tuesday following my end-of-the-world party, I'm in a therapy session with Veronica, and I feel that contraction — the stifling sense of being boxed in. Each time I drink, I can feel the very essence of who I am disappearing from view. I already know the answer, but I plead with Veronica to guide me. She responds with her usual quiet steadiness, reminding me she would never tell me what to do, but that she does have a question for me to consider: 'Is drinking getting you closer to the life you want, or further away?'

In that moment, the instinct that's been chipping away at me in fevered whispers breaks through my unconscious and is now standing front and centre, too loud to ignore. I know then that sobriety is the next and necessary step towards the life I've always imagined for myself. One that is big and bright and bold and unafraid. It won't be easy, but I'm sure in every cell of my being that it's the right decision.

This time, I don't make a public announcement. No social media confessionals or soul-bearing blog posts. I just quietly tell my closest friends I've decided to quit drinking. I don't set a time limit. It might be a month; it might be forever. I just know that the blurred view that comes with alcohol no longer serves me, and that I need to see what lies beyond.

I stumble across an image by artist Samuel Leighton-Dore that sums up what this process means to me. On the left, he has drawn an iceberg. Visible above the water on the iceberg's crest are a collection of words in jagged boxes: *anger; habits; fear; ideas; addictions; shame.* Underneath the water, the iceberg is bigger and deeper, a pointed tip extending into the depths of the ocean. On this part, the boxes read: *self aversion; rejection; childhood traumas; hurt that you thought you'd deal with; times you were humiliated; the ways you changed when you didn't belong; your nervous system being wired to panic; the way you were.* Pointing to the iceberg with an arrow is the word *you*. To the right of the image is a small yellow submarine moving towards the iceberg, with a face visible through a small, round window. Pointing to the submarine is the word *therapy*.

How neatly this encapsulates the work we do in therapy — the exhumation of past hurt hidden deep beneath the surface. But it's a caption that Samuel writes when he reposts the image on Instagram after his own decision to stop drinking that knocks the wind out of me. He writes: 'If therapy is the yellow submarine, sobriety is defrosting the little round window and being strapped to the seat, with nowhere to divert your eyes.' Ooft.

Therapy is a deep dive to all the places that scare me. And yet I often can't bear to look at what I uncover. Alcohol is fogging up that little window. On 28 June 2019, I decide to give sobriety another go. This is my chance to demist the glass. Time to hold the wounds up to the light and to let the healing begin.

* * *

IT'S EMPOWERING TO say goodbye to hangovers and to embrace Sunday mornings again. Almost immediately, I start to feel better. My moods stabilise, and I no longer feel like I'm trapped in a pinball machine, careening from crisis to recovery and back again. I'm eager to gain a deeper understanding of the impact alcohol is having on my mental health, in the hope it will provide convincing reasons not to go back. I'd skirted around the edges of this in my first year of sobriety, but perhaps wasn't brave enough to explore it in depth. This time, I'm ready to do the work. I know on the most rudimentary level that drinking affects your mood, but I hadn't fully grasped just how risky it was for someone like me, with a brain predisposed to panic.

I begin to read widely — dipping into the vast canon of 'quit lit' that has emerged since my first year off the booze. These are books similar to *High Sobriety*, written largely by women like me, who were good-time party girls trapped in a noxious relationship with alcohol. Many discuss the impact that binge drinking was having on their mental health, and how sobriety helped turn it around. For so long, I thought there was something unique and unusual about the hangxiety I felt after a big night on the piss — or, increasingly as I got older, after just a couple of glasses of wine. I thought it was merely another fun side effect of a life lived in a state of high anxiety. But the more I read these women's stories, the more apparent it becomes that this dreadful feeling of agitation and high-octane panic is not an anomaly familiar only to my misbehaving brain, but a fundamental hallmark of the average hangover.

I delve into the science, and what I find is both comforting and confronting. When you wake up blanketed in a catastrophic cloud of doom that leaves you questioning every decision you've made since you were old enough to talk, it's not happening by accident. If you feel like you're having a mental breakdown after a night of drinking, that's because essentially you are. Your body and mind are in withdrawal from alcohol, and that sets off a chain of events that can create absolute pandemonium. It's a chemical storm in your brain.

Alcohol targets two brain receptors that send messages to our nervous system. The first, gaba, is an inhibitor, which calms us down. Then there's glutamate, which has the opposite effect, exciting the brain. When we drink, it stimulates gaba and blocks glutamate, making us feel temporarily warm and fuzzy, prompting us to lose inhibitions and express our undying love to randoms at parties. For those prone to anxiety, it can temporarily turn down the chatter in an over-stimulated mind. But when we wake up the next morning, the brain registers that this is not the natural order of things, and tries to correct itself. It floods your nervous system with glutamate and blocks gaba, the calming chemical. It's like a car with a stuck accelerator and no brakes. You feel agitated and restless because your brain is in overdrive.

I also learn that being hungover stimulates the release of cortisol and noradrenaline — the body's fight-or-flight hormones, which can exacerbate anxious feelings. Then there's the disrupted sleep. It's harder to reach the REM stage of the sleep cycle after a big boozy night, which means you miss out on the part that helps the brain rest and rejuvenate. You don't have to have a pre-existing mental health condition to feel the impact of all this, but it's likely to be amplified in those already struggling. The more I understand about alcohol's impact on the brain, the harder it is to ignore the incontrovertible truth — drinking when you have chronic anxiety is like pouring petrol on a bonfire and watching your life blow up around you.

And yet, one of the great lies propagated by popular culture and a shrewd alcohol industry is that drinking helps us cope. Having a tough day? Sink a refreshing beer. Life falling apart? Pour yourself a glass of Pinot — you've earned it. For me, it was always a short-term burst of escapism, swiftly followed by an emotional arse-kicking. I'd often drink to numb pain, only to have the pain rebound ten-fold the next day. Then I'd drink again, just so I didn't have to feel the stuff that this numbing agent was meant to block out but had only amplified. It's only during my second go at sobriety that I see just how illogical and self-destructive this cycle has become. Alcohol is a terrible therapist, and a capricious friend. Rather than pouring accelerant on the bonfire, I need to start lighting myself up from the inside and build a life I don't need to escape from.

This is something that Holly Whitaker talks about in her book, *Quit Like a Woman*. She writes: 'The achievement of sobriety is not the point; it's a by-product of the work. The work is the point … sobriety is the catalyst to heal deeper wounds.'

This time around, I can see that cutting out alcohol is only the start of the journey. Sobriety doesn't remove your problems — it reveals them. You can see in full focus the issues that need your attention. And, all too often, those issues are shrouded in shame. We reach for a glass of wine to counter the shame of feeling we're not good enough, to forget painful memories, or to paper over the discomfort of not fitting in or being as confident as we'd like. Then we wake up with a hangover, disgusted with ourselves for repeating the same drunken mistakes and not being able to drink in moderation.

Shame can be corrosive. It doesn't motivate us to change — it leaves us paralysed by guilt and inertia. The human brain likes familiarity. There can be comfort and safety in repeating the same patterns, even if they're bad for us.

Not being able to drink like a 'normal' person has been a source of great shame for me. I don't identify as an alcoholic, but I know I'm not the kind of person who can stop at one glass. What I hadn't considered is that few people can. This product I've been trying so hard to use moderately is one of the five most addictive substances in the world — up there with heroin, cocaine, barbiturates, and nicotine — and by its very chemical nature is designed to keep us wanting more.

As Ruby Warrington proposes in *Sober Curious*, anyone who drinks alcohol on a regular basis is 'a little bit addicted'. Some may be further down the path than others, but Warrington believes the fact we're biologically hardwired to seek out more alcohol, because it artificially stimulates the brain's pleasure circuity — coupled with the way we're marketed booze from an early age as a necessary part of social bonding — makes it almost impossible to drink in moderation. And yet, so many of us beat ourselves up for being stuck in a cycle of binge drinking, viewing it as a moral failing rather than the logical outcome of regularly consuming a highly addictive substance that is so foreign to our bodies we use it to fuel our cars.

Taking off the cloak of shame, I can see that it was almost inevitable I'd return to old habits after my initial year of sobriety, and that moderation is a battle most drinkers can't win. I know only a handful of people who can easily stop after one. Drinking is not only socially accepted — it's socially expected. Perhaps my shame does not belong with me, but with an alcohol industry that tries to convince us this highly dangerous drug is a benign substance. Alcohol is the only drug we have to justify not taking. But the stigma around dependency remains. Sobriety is often perceived as a weakness. If you have to stop drinking completely, you must lack self-control — the irony being that many people casting these judgments consume alcohol so regularly they couldn't fathom surviving a social situation without it. They're the same people who ask, 'Why can't you just have one or two?' as they drain their sixth glass of wine.

I choose abstinence because it's easier than moderation. Putting boundaries around my drinking — only at weekends, not after 10.00 p.m., alternating every second drink with water — is too much effort. The mental gymnastics required to constantly bargain with yourself over a substance that will always have the upper hand is exhausting. Sometimes, for the life you want, you have to sacrifice the short-term fix for a greater reward.

Several months into quitting drinking, and the rewards are plentiful. My Mood Flow diary is a sea of pink. There is still some beige — because life will always be a bit meh from time to time — but the blue and dark-blue days have all but disappeared. In therapy, I'm able to tackle issues that had previously felt too confronting. I'm going deep into the core of those complex fears, flaws, and foibles, and gaining a full and clear picture of myself. That little window in the submarine has been defogged, and I'm finally looking at what lies on the other side. It's challenging, but it's also liberating. I understand myself better, and like myself more. That makes the tough days easier to bear.

It quickly becomes apparent that after therapy, sobriety is the single most effective step I've taken for my mental health. It's not that I don't struggle. But when the road gets rocky, I don't fall down as hard or for as long as I once did. I'm not avoiding uncomfortable emotions; I'm facing them head on. Removing alcohol has stripped me bare. There's nowhere left to hide. But although I uncover some pain and discomfort, what I didn't expect to find was a deep well of strength and resilience. I'm not sure I would have found that, had I kept drinking. I'm proud I got to this place. It feels like nothing could knock me off the course.

Unprecedented

IT'S EARLY MARCH 2020, and I'm on stage at the Sydney Opera House — one of the world's most famous landmarks. It's a real 'pinch me' moment. I'm appearing as a guest of the All About Women festival, on a 'Sober Curious' panel moderated by feminist author Clementine Ford, and featuring TV host and author Yumi Stynes, and Shanna Whan, founder of bush charity, Sober in the Country. I talk about the rewards of sobriety, the strength I feel at my core, but also the sense of loss that comes from letting go of your old life. I'm asked by an audience member if there's a grief that accompanies sobriety, and I admit that when I realised I would probably never get drunk again, I was sad. I grieved for those late-night adventures, the spontaneity and the silliness. And I mourned the part of myself I was losing — Starkers, the party girl, who was being placed into early retirement. But I tell the questioner that whenever I get misty-eyed about the fun times, I think about where those drunken nights would take me. I can't just freeze-frame the good bits — I have to play the tape forward. And when I do, I see the drunken mishaps and injuries, the blackouts and strained relationships, the crashing mental health, and the weeks of self-loathing. I'm not sad to farewell that.

Afterwards, I walk back to my hotel to get my bag before heading to the airport. It's been 19 years since I first arrived in Sydney as a wide-eyed backpacker on the first stop of my tour around Australia. I spent a riotous first week partying until dawn with new friends from all over the world and sleeping off the hangovers in a musty hostel dorm. My life looks markedly different today, but one thing remains constant — the harbour view and its power to take my breath away.

Docked on the opposite side of the harbour is a huge cruise ship. It's as tall as an apartment block. I gaze at it, dumbfounded by the size of the thing, wondering how it remains upright on the water. It's called the *Ruby Princess*. Within weeks, this name will become seared into the Australian public's consciousness. Hitching a ride with the grey nomads on this floating hotel is a virus that will bring the world shuddering to a stop.

Prior to my Sydney trip, I was aware of something called Covid-19, which had originated in China and was being talked up as a contagion that could have catastrophic global implications. But as a former tabloid journalist well-versed in the art of hyperbole, my cynicism bred a complacent ignorance. On the list of things my anxious brain was prone to worry about, a once-in-a-century pandemic hadn't even registered in the top hundred.

Back in Melbourne, things escalate quickly. What had seemed a vague and distant threat is suddenly a real and present danger. There are chaotic scenes outside the gates of the Australian Grand Prix on the morning of Friday 13 March, as furious racegoers queuing to enter the track are informed by a man holding a loudhailer that the event has been called off. One after another, statements are issued by the organisers of major events, regretfully cancelling plans. The Melbourne International Comedy Festival; the Food and Wine Festival; a Robbie Williams stadium gig; the Melbourne Fashion Festival — a series of dominoes falling, each one adding to the foreboding sense that something uniquely terrible is unfolding. Over the next two years we will long for a return to precedented times.

In Italy, parts of the country are already in lockdown, the health system is buckling, and deaths are rising. This, the medical experts in Australia warn, is a portent of what we face if drastic steps are not taken. Amid the confusion and heightened anxiety, Australia's prime minister, Scott Morrison, holds a press conference, announcing that all non-essential gatherings of more than 500 people will be banned from Monday, and then inexplicably declares he'll still go to the footy on Saturday night to watch his rugby league team, the Sharks, because, 'it might be the last chance for a while'.

The next few weeks go past in a blur. I flinch at headlines of corpses piling up in Italian morgues, the elderly dying in alarming numbers. Australia has already placed a travel ban on China and Italy, and there is talk of international borders being closed completely. The situation in the UK is deteriorating, and I start panicking about my parents in Scotland, spending a tearful phone call with my brother debating whether to get on a plane home to Edinburgh before it's too late. We decide I should stay where I am, my parents assuring me that they'll be following government 'shielding' advice for over-70s to stay home and avoid face-to-face contact for at least 12 weeks.

On 20 March 2020, Australia closes its international borders, not only barring foreign nationals from entering, but becoming one of the few countries in the world to place a ban on its own citizens from leaving. The border will remain closed for almost two years. It will be the longest time I've ever been separated from my family.

A national lockdown is being discussed, and it appears inevitable we'll follow much of the world and shut down the country to try to slow the spread of the virus. There is panic buying in supermarkets. A toilet roll becomes the hottest commodity. I send myself a cake, and spend my 44th birthday at home alone, playing games with my friends through an app called House Party. Nothing about this situation is normal. There are no reference points to guide us. It's the most bewildering, foreign experience.

It's only been nine months since I quit drinking. I wrestle with the urge to get back on it. If you can't have a wine in the middle of a global pandemic, when can you? I'm no longer sober-curious — I'm shit-faced–curious. I want to know what it would be like to drink myself into oblivion while the world crumbles around me.

I'm not alone. Long queues start forming at bottle shops. It's unclear which industries will be shut down, and there is growing angst that access to booze will be curtailed. In the end, alcohol retailers are deemed an 'essential service' and allowed to keep trading. But in a move offering a frightening glimpse into what's considered a normal level of alcohol consumption in this country, major chains impose limits to prevent stockpiling — two cases (a case being 24 cans) of beer, cider, or premixed spirits, 12 bottles of wine, and two bottles of spirits per purchase.

On 31 March, we enter a national lockdown. We have only four permitted reasons to leave the house — for food and supplies, for exercise, for medical care, or for work and education if deemed essential. The pace at which our world has been upended is dizzying. Overnight, we have been untethered from all the pillars of our lives that anchored us.

As someone who lives alone, I wonder how I will survive being confined to my home without company for what the prime minister says will be six weeks, but also warns could be as long as six months. I love living alone, but ordinarily I get to choose when I have company. Now, my only human contact will be meeting up with a friend for a socially distanced walk. The thought of not being able to physically touch another person for months leaves me bereft. We were not designed to live like this.

In the week before lockdown, spending at liquor stores rises by 86 per cent. Health experts warn that a perfect storm is brewing, as those already vulnerable to the harms of heavy drinking now face the stress of lockdown and the potential loss of work while having all constraints on their drinking habits removed. It's easier to drink during the day when you have no job to go to, or you can work from home hungover or tipsy and not have to face your boss in person. Friends start joking about having 'breakfast beers' because, fuck it, why not?

I think about what my alcohol consumption would look like if I wasn't already sober. Would I be sneaking wines in between Zoom meetings? If previous habits are any indicator, the answer is probably yes. It doesn't take long to lose the desire to seek solace at the bottom of a glass. These are indeed unprecedented times; I'll need every ounce of resilience to see me through. The only thing worse than raging hangxiety would be raging hangxiety while trapped in your apartment alone for weeks on end as a deadly virus decimates the planet.

I decide that if alcohol is the answer, I'm asking the wrong question. Instead, I ponder what I'll need to keep me afloat in these uncharted waters. One of the hardest things to navigate is the ceaseless uncertainty. We have no idea what's coming next, how this will end, or what state we'll be in when it does. Rather than give in to helplessness, I create pockets of certainty throughout my day — little islands of sanity that I can cling to as proof that some things remain in my control. My routine includes a lunchtime walk, connecting with a friend on the phone or FaceTime, and ending my working day with a self-isolation dance party for one, where I turn on disco lights, crank up my favourite cheesy pop tunes, and let loose in my lounge room until I've sweated out the anxious energy.

After a few weeks, a calm descends. My shoulders drop and the tension melts away as I surrender to a scaled-back version of my normal life. My world has shrunk, but so too has my anxiety. Life in lockdown is simple. It's less frantic and reduced to the basics: eat, sleep, walk, work, take time to connect with the people I love. In some ways, people who have lived with anxiety for years are the experts for these times. If you spend your whole life worrying about the day that might never happen, when that day actually comes, you're ready. I know how to survive when stability has gone and the life you once knew has become a shape-shifting beast you don't recognise anymore. These are the times when you have to reduce your existence to the most rudimentary goals, take each hour at a time, and celebrate every small win.

I'm also grateful to have a safe place to call home, and secure work. I took a voluntary redundancy from *The Age* in 2016, and since then have enjoyed a portfolio career, taking on a steady stream of contract and freelance work as a speechwriter, journalist, mental health advocate, content creator, public speaker, and media consultant in the not-for-profit, media, and mental health sectors. Despite the economic downturn, I'm relieved that the work continues to come in. The psychological fallout of a global pandemic is profound and far-reaching, and the demand for mental health content skyrockets, keeping me busy. The work acts as an anchor, both financially and emotionally.

With fewer social pressures on my time, the chatter in my head grows quieter. The niggling FOMO (fear of missing out), which often meant my diary was crammed with events, is gone. It's comforting knowing that all over the world, people are staying home, just like me. Time spent with friends and family — whether on Zoom or on a neighbourhood walk — is becoming more meaningful. I'm more present, and appreciate the simple privilege of being loved and valued by people who you love back. The 'always on' culture that left me overwhelmed and over-scheduled is exposed by this enforced slowdown as an unhealthy trap. I lean into the stillness while it lasts.

But my calmness is also a product of my sobriety. Since I quit drinking, I've felt something slowly building inside me. It's a profound connection to the person I had lost underneath the noise, drama, and social conditioning that came with drinking. I'm developing a strength at my core I'd forgotten was there. Being in touch with that side of myself feels life-giving. The crisis we're living through is infinitely more manageable because I'm not drinking. I'm not having to contend with the rollercoaster of mood dips or waking up dusty with all the problems of the world magnified. Throwing alcohol into the mix of this incredibly difficult year is unimaginable. I just don't think I'd survive it.

When the six-week lockdown is over, we tentatively return to our old lives, albeit a scaled-back version that still restricts how we work, socialise, and move around. But our hard-earned freedoms are short-lived. By the beginning of July, Melbourne is back in lockdown, and will remain that way for four months. While the rest of the country returns to some semblance of normality, Victoria is declared a state of disaster as the virus takes hold again and we enter harsh stage-four restrictions. We're only permitted to leave home for an hour each day for exercise, and are confined to a five-kilometre radius, with a nightly curfew from 8.00 p.m. to 5.00 a.m. It's gruelling. Living alone becomes a huge challenge. I start to long for the touch of another human. Just someone to sit on the couch with and debrief. Someone to hold me when I feel unsteady. The experts call this 'skin hunger' — a primal need for physical connection. The video calls that once sustained me now feel like a cruel and hollow imitation of intimacy. I just want to hug my mum.

It will be ten weeks before the government recognises the mental health impacts of prolonged isolation for people living alone and allows us to nominate one person with whom we can form a 'single social bubble' and receive home visits. Having my best friend, Jason, come over a couple of times a week feels like being thrown a life raft.

Melbourne will eventually earn the ignominious title of the most locked-down city in the world, enduring 263 days over six lockdowns in 2020 and 2021. There are times when it feels as if this strange state of suspended animation will never end. But my commitment to my sobriety doesn't falter. It's one of the reasons I'm not falling apart. And yet everywhere I turn, I'm bombarded with advertising that tells me drinking is my best survival tool. During lockdown, an industry not known for its social responsibility abandons any pretence of being a good corporate citizen, and starts to use this public health crisis as a marketing tool. It's aggressive, targeted, and relentless.

A survey by the Foundation for Alcohol Research and Education (FARE) finds that in just one hour on a Friday night in the first lockdown, 107 sponsored alcohol advertisements are displayed on the average person's Facebook and Instagram accounts — approximately one every 35 seconds. Key marketing messages include getting easy access to alcohol without leaving your home, and drinking to cope, survive, or feel better about isolation and the pandemic. With phrases such as 'Stay in. Drink up' and 'confinement sale', it's not even subtle.

The messaging is brutally effective. Sales of home-delivered alcohol skyrocket, and one in five Australian households report buying more than usual during lockdown. And in those households, 70 per cent of people report they're drinking more than they did before Covid hit. More than one-third of all those surveyed by FARE are now drinking daily, and say they're concerned with the amount of alcohol they or someone they live with is drinking. Twenty-eight per cent say they're drinking to cope with anxiety and stress, and 20 per cent are drinking earlier in the day.

My old mate Chris Raine, founder of Hello Sunday Morning — which has now grown to an organisation with global reach — reports a significant increase in people registering for their Daybreak app, a tool to help people cut back on alcohol or quit drinking altogether. Lockdown has created the perfect conditions to habituate people to drinking daily. He tells *The Guardian* it can have a cascading effect, where weekend drinkers become weekday drinkers, social drinkers become daily drinkers, and those at the acute end, who were wrestling with addiction and relied on face-to-face support from groups such as Alcoholics Anonymous to stay sober, are at risk of relapse.

The queues at bottle shops before lockdown were indicative, Chris says, of a culture that sees alcohol as an 'essential medicine'. Authorities had no choice but to exempt alcohol retailers from shutdowns, because doing otherwise would be unthinkable. 'You'd have tens of thousands of people going into involuntary detox and not having the health system able to cope. I wish people didn't culturally depend on alcohol the way we do.'

This dependency remains a feature of Melbourne's lockdowns, and is reinforced by messaging that goes right to the top of government. At the start of the pandemic, when Victorian premier Dan Andrews tells a rattled community that pubs will close, he warns, 'That doesn't mean you can have all your mates around to your home and get on the beers.' The phrase is mashed up into a song with some heavy electronic beats, and becomes a cult classic. Andrews, who fronts a press conference for 120 consecutive days, is repeatedly asked when it will be time to 'get on the beers'. We're all craving a return to more familiar times, and the message we're given is that life will be normal again when we can drink.

On 26 October, the premier addresses the media once more. His voice breaking with emotion, he tells the people of his exhausted state that the 16-week lockdown will end. I watch it live, and it's like a dam wall breaking. The fear and frustration; the persistent low hum of anxiety; the grief and the uncertainty, and the bone-crushing loneliness — it all comes crashing over me, and I sob. You don't realise how tightly you've been holding on until you finally loosen your grip.

Andrews is asked by a reporter whether he'd be 'getting on the beers'. He quips, 'I don't know that I'll be drinking a beer tonight: I might go a little higher up the shelf.' He's roundly applauded for his response. I get it. After months of dashed hopes, bracing ourselves to expect the worst as an act of self-preservation, people are entitled to some light relief. But it lands uncomfortably for me. It makes me want a drink in a way I haven't for a long time. Not because I think it will make me happier — life is calmer and more fulfilling since I chose sobriety — but because drinking is being sold as the essential bonding experience to mark the end of a period that has been so scarring. It feels alienating to hear 'get on the beers' embraced as cultural shorthand for belonging. And it troubles me that the way we're being encouraged to process our collective trauma is by getting drunk.

My first dinner out with girlfriends is surreal and somewhat of a sensory overload. It feels like we're emerging blinking into the light after a prolonged hibernation. Being thrust back into a noisy world of colour and movement feels foreign and exhausting, but it's so good to be together again with people I love. We dine at a French restaurant, and I call ahead to ask if I can bring non-alcoholic champagne. Their menu offers little for the non-drinker, and I want to share the sense of occasion with my friends as we celebrate the end of a period that will stay with us forever. The restaurant agrees, but I'm charged $14 corkage — almost twice as much as the wine itself. When the waitress brings my friends' wine over, she looks at me pityingly, joking that I'm 'being punished' — the implication being that not being able to drink alcohol is the greatest deprivation. I force a laugh, but it irritates me. The only punishing thing about this scenario is being alienated for your sobriety.

As the weather warms up and the 'get on the beers' narrative continues apace, TV networks do live crosses from beer gardens to illustrate our return to normality. It's tricky terrain for me to traverse, but I'm proud I continue to have the courage to swim against the social tide. It doesn't take long to find my rhythm and to settle back into sober socialising. The more events I attend without alcohol, the more I'm reminded I don't need a drink to have fun or to be myself.

We enjoy a few months of relative freedom as restrictions ease, and I feel so grateful for the little things I'd missed: a weekend down the coast with friends; swimming in the ocean; brunch in my favourite cafe; the ability to leave the house without a permitted reason.

On New Year's Eve, I go to a party, and dance and laugh and drink non-alcoholic beers and hug my friends. I don't miss drinking at all. I enjoy being present with the people I love, and relish knowing that I can drive myself home at 1.00 a.m. and wake up the next day without regrets. In the morning, it's a beautiful New Year's Day, and I go for a long walk in the sunshine around Princes Park, where all those years ago I made the decision to give alcohol a break while battling the worst hangover of my life. I think about how far I've come and the year I've survived, and find myself in tears. Happy tears. Grateful tears. Living through a pandemic has brought times of anxiety, loss, and loneliness, but there were also many moments of connection, community, and gratitude for the simplest pleasures. While I was separated from the people who mean the most to me, the extraordinary nature of the obstacles we've faced has meant I have loved and been loved more deeply than perhaps I ever have. This past year has taught me that you can't take anything for granted. If yesterday is gone and tomorrow isn't guaranteed, the only moment you have is right now.

I reflect on the strength it took to keep pushing through the more challenging parts of this extremely challenging period in human history, and my heart swells with pride to think I did it without alcohol. Then I feel it again — that deep connection to the part of me that is resilient and vibrant and untethered from the need to follow the pack to fit in. What joy there is in truly knowing yourself. And being proud of the person you find when you have the courage to peel back the layers. I'm grateful for the life I'm building.

The freedoms are sweet, but they don't last. By February, we're back in lockdown. This time, just for five days. But then May comes, and we're back in for a fortnight. By winter, it's groundhog day as we enter another lockdown, and then another long and gruelling one that lasts for three months. Through it all, I'm again grateful for my sobriety, and it helps stabilise me when we have to contend with not only our sixth lockdown, but violent anti-vaxxer riots in Melbourne's CBD, and even a 5.8 magnitude earthquake.

I decide to share what I'm learning from this alcohol-free life, launching #NoBoozeDayTuesday on my Instagram page, where every Tuesday I invite people to take one night off drinking and join me online as I answer questions on sobriety. I'm inundated with people grappling with their drinking. Lockdown has been so hard, and some have been using alcohol to stay afloat. Only now they're realising that their life raft is a dead weight pulling them under.

We finally emerge from lockdown on 22 October 2021. I don't think anyone in Melbourne will ever be the same again. Some bring with them baggage that will take a long time to unpack. The Alcohol and Drug Foundation finds that 25 per cent of Australians are drinking more than they did before the pandemic, to cope with stress and anxiety, including 58 per cent of households with children. Demand for alcohol and other drug services increases substantially. In 2021, Australians make more than 25,000 calls to the National Alcohol and Other Drug Hotline — triple the pre-pandemic numbers of 2019.

The most impacted are women aged between their 40s and 60s. Rehab clinicians say women who were social drinkers prior to the pandemic have transitioned to drinking at home, often alone, and are using alcohol as a form of self-soothing to manage family and financial pressures exacerbated by the loss of social connection that came with lockdown.

Throughout the pandemic, women — who are more likely to work in casualised industries — are over-represented in job losses, and they shoulder a disproportionate share of unpaid care, home schooling, and household labour, so it's perhaps not surprising they'd be more at risk of developing risky drinking habits.

But for many people — not just women — lockdown is a circuit breaker. It forces them to confront the way they drink, and offers an opportunity to change course. For those looking for a new direction, they're reaching it at just the right time. The pandemic accelerates a trend that was already gathering pace. This period of great disruption gives rise to a shift in social norms that will subvert the drinking culture as we know it. Being sober is about to get a whole lot easier.

Sober revolution

THROUGHOUT MY SOBER journey, it's often struck me that it's not my sobriety that's challenging, but society's reaction to it. How different things could be if not-drinking was normalised — if sober customers were treated with the same respect as drinkers, and were given more options. Then, in the middle of the pandemic, something unexpected happens. A non-alcoholic beer, Heaps Normal, is launched. It's not the first, but there's something about this one that cuts through and thrusts sobriety into the mainstream. Right name, right time, right market. It quickly starts outselling regular beer in many bottle shops — a trend that takes everyone by surprise. Around the same time, several online and shopfront non-alcoholic bottle shops open, meeting the growing demand for alcohol-free products. And in between Melbourne lockdowns, Australia's first non-alcoholic bar, Brunswick Aces, opens its doors in a flurry of national publicity. I'm reminded of the Australian Hotels Association representative who told me, during my first stint off the booze, that a pub that doesn't serve beer or liquor would be 'odd' and that he couldn't think 'why on earth it would work here in Australia'.

It's gratifying to see how wrong he was. The rise of the 'non-alc' drinks category in recent years is nothing short of stratospheric, and mirrors the growing popularity of sobriety. What was once a niche area of drinks that felt like pale, watery imitations of the real thing is now a booming business sector with increasingly sophisticated beers, wines, and spirits, which have often undergone the same complex and careful distillation processes as alcoholic drinks. In the 12 months to May 2021, liquor giants BWS and Dan Murphy's report sales of non-alcoholic drinks have more than doubled, while some smaller chains are seeing growth of more than 200 per cent. After launching in July 2020, Heaps Normal is now a $58 million business with more than 4,000 wholesale customers, and joins a booming low- and no-alcohol category that drinks-market-analysis company IWSR projects will grow by 31 per cent by 2024.

It's taken a while to get here, but Australia is catching up with a trend that has been underway overseas for years. At an investor relations day, Japanese brewer Asahi reports that the growth of alcoholic beverages is flat, but that the worldwide growth of products with less than 0.1 per cent of alcohol by volume is close to 6 per cent.

Heaps Normal was created by four Aussie friends — Peter Brennan, Andy Miller, Ben Holdstock, and Jordy Smith — so their mates could feel proud taking to a barbecue 'something that didn't scream "I'm sober."' They believe their success is part of a non-alcoholic counter-culture that has been simmering away for some time. 'People are more conscious about what they're putting into their bodies these days, and the whole health and wellness movement is really starting to pop,' Brennan tells me. 'When I was 15, we'd drink anything — a two-litre bottle of white lightning [cider] — and think we were heroes because we were taught that you drink for any occasion, and that's normal. Our mission as a business is questioning normal, and changing the drinking culture. But we've never preached sobriety, and that's probably helped us because we're not demonising alcohol.'

The clever positioning of their brand as one that can be enjoyed by those who drink and those who are sober, with the tagline 'too good to be wasted', speaks to a community with an increasing thirst for moderation and abstinence, and looking for a cool alternative to alcohol. Sobriety is being heaps normalised.

Drinks like this weren't widely available the first time I quit drinking, so discovering them is a game-changer. They allow me to take part in the ritual and ceremony of drinking without all the drama that alcohol brings. I can enjoy a cold beer on a hot day at a backyard barbecue, and still stay sober. I start to seek out bars that offer appealing non-alcoholic options, and am heartened to notice that venues with few or no alcohol-free alternatives are becoming the exception, not the norm. On Instagram, I find myself gravitating towards the growing number of accounts championing the push for more alcohol-free beverages in the hospitality industry and brands selling enticing non-alcoholic beer, wines, and spirits. While once I was despairing at the soda water-and-lime offerings being served up, there are now so many choices that I can even turn to 'sober sommeliers' to help me curate my own dynamic zero-alcohol drinks list.

But there is tension within sober circles about whether drinks that smell, look, and taste like alcohol might act as a gateway back to alcohol for those grappling with dependency. The first time I tried an alcohol-free beer, I felt that buzz within minutes. There was a head rush, and my whole body tingled. How powerful the placebo effect must be that this drink, which was almost a perfect imitation of real beer, made my brain believe I was drunk. The feeling quickly subsided, but I could see why some have concerns about these drinks being sold in supermarkets next to bottled water. The counter-argument is that it's safer for someone with a history of alcohol abuse to get their non-alcoholic drinks while buying groceries than it would be to walk into a bottle shop.

Given the alcohol industry's chequered history of actively

causing social harm, I'm sceptical of the liquor giants' expansion into the non-alcoholic space. When Dan Murphy's announces it will launch a pop-up alcohol-free bar in Melbourne's well-to-do bayside suburbs in March 2022 — almost a year after Brunswick Aces opens its doors — I can't help but feel it's little more than a marketing stunt to get people talking about their brand. This is the same company that recently dragged an Aboriginal community through the courts, fighting to open a cut-price liquor barn in a dry area, despite Indigenous elders pleading that problem drinking was already so high it would cause profound damage. This sudden interest in 'changing the drinking culture' seems to me like Big Tobacco sponsoring a cancer ward.

The major chains may be cashing in on the growing demand for non-alcoholic options, but there's no doubt they'll be concerned about their bottom line if it continues. A study by the Centre for Alcohol Policy Research, released in March 2022, shows that just 5 per cent of the population drink more than a third of all alcohol consumed in Australia — on average, almost eight drinks a day. The heaviest drinking 20 per cent account for 75 per cent of all alcohol consumed. For an industry reliant on problem drinkers to survive, the march of the sober-curious movement is an existential threat.

But it's a trend that shows no sign of abating. The pandemic has turbocharged a change in the nation's drinking habits. Perhaps it's unsurprising that a seismic event that is rocking the foundations of our very existence would concentrate the mind on the meaning of life and the way we're living it. If life is short, and you never know what's around the corner, why waste it being hungover? It's interesting that this shift is being led by young people. The binge-drinking generation, which experts once warned me is an alcohol timebomb waiting to go off, is slowing down.

The most recent National Drug Strategy Household survey — released every three years, and considered the most reliable indicator of trends in alcohol consumption — shows that between 2001 and 2019, harmful drinking remained stable for older Australians, but significantly decreased in younger age groups. The proportion of 18- to 24-year-olds drinking in ways that put them at lifetime risk dropped from 31 per cent to 18.8 per cent. And the proportion putting themselves at risk on a single occasion of drinking, on at least a monthly basis, dropped from 57 per cent to 41 per cent. The number of people in this age group abstaining altogether rose from 9.7 per cent to 21 per cent.

The age at which young people have their first drink is also changing. The number of teenagers aged 14 to 17 who have never consumed alcohol rose from 28 per cent in 2001 to 66 per cent in 2019. It's a trend replicated in many countries, and is reflected in the changing face of those seeking support from Hello Sunday Morning. While younger people are drinking less, their parents and grandparents are entering the latter stages of their lives with problematic drinking habits.

In 2010, when Hello Sunday Morning began, most people registering were in their early 20s. Now the average age is 47. Almost 80 per cent of their 115,000 users are aged between 35 and 70. Sixty-six per cent are women, many of whom are working mothers, juggling mid-life stresses such as relationship challenges, financial difficulties, family dynamics, and ageing parents.

But there is a mood for change among this cohort, reflected in the huge boom in sobriety coaches — often middle-aged women who have quit drinking and have lessons to share with women like them. They commonly specialise in what's called 'grey area' drinking — catering for those who land somewhere between a fall-down drunk and an occasional tippler who drinks one glass of Prosecco at Christmas but is mostly abstinent. Again, it's a smart shift in messaging that allows people who have a problematic dependence on alcohol, but don't feel the need to join Alcoholics Anonymous, to seek support without the shame of being branded an addict.

The next national alcohol-consumption statistics were due in early 2023, which would give an indication of what, if any, lasting impact Covid has had on Australian drinking patterns. But, anecdotally, the trend of younger people drinking less has continued beyond the height of the pandemic. Findings from a survey released by Drinkwise in July 2021 found that Australians aged 18 to 44 are twice as likely to consume zero-alcohol and low-strength alcohol drinks as those aged over 45. And in November the same year, at schoolies — the once-drunken rite of passage for school leavers partying at beachside resorts to mark the end of their final high school exams — Gold Coast police say attendees 'aren't as drunk as they used to be'. The number of teenagers receiving emergency ambulance treatment has halved, they say, and the crowd is the most well behaved they've had in five years.

Researchers say the reasons for young people's changing drinking patterns are complex. The threat of climate change, the rising cost of living, and being reliant on renting indefinitely make for an uncertain future, leaving many with a need to gain control over their lives. Being raised in a digital age has also bred wariness about putting images on social media that could impact their job prospects in an already volatile employment market. And they're more health conscious than their parents' generation, perhaps having heeded the public health messages directed at them that began in 2008 with then prime minister Kevin Rudd's national binge-drinking strategy, which I covered during my time reporting on alcohol issues for *The Age*. These days, getting blind drunk is not seen as accumulating the same social capital as it once did.

But perhaps the biggest change is that young people are coming of age at a time when moderation or abstinence is being reframed as a source of pride, not shame Social media were once blamed for normalising binge drinking, with young people boasting online about their huge nights on the piss; now the social-contagion effect is now operating in reverse, and social media are being used to celebrate healthy living and sobriety. In the last decade, there has been a boom in online communities, podcasts, books, and even 'conscious clubbing' dance parties that celebrate the sober lifestyle. On Instagram and TikTok, a growing cohort of vibrant young influencers living their best lives without alcohol are offering a compelling counterargument to the perception that sobriety equals social suicide.

Groups such as Sober Girls Society, Hip Sobriety, It's Not Me it's Booze, Sober Evolution, Club Soda, Soberistas, The Mindful Mocktail, and Sexy Sobriety have created fun, welcoming spaces for the sober or sober-curious to feel inspired and empowered. For those who want more hands-on, scientific support, groups such as This Naked Mind, Hello Sunday Morning, and Tempest offer a judgement-free space to understand drinking habits and change unhealthy patterns.

This rich vein of research and peer support has made my second crack at sobriety much less isolating. The sober community gives me a chance to connect with people who experience the same highs and lows of alcohol-free living. Through Australian online group Sober Mates, I meet founder Sam Wilson, a 28-year-old former 'heavy social drinker' who quit alcohol at 26, just before the pandemic hit, and is now a walking, talking billboard for the wild and rich existence you can have when you show up fully present in your own life. She is one of the most effervescent people I've ever met, and credits sobriety with her newfound confidence on the dating scene, buying her own apartment, and enthusiastically meeting the dawn with ocean swims and invigorating ice baths. 'My world was really closing in when I was drinking. Now I've got so much energy and space, and my whole world has opened up,' she says. 'The best compliment I've had was a friend who said I was living life for me.

That's what sobriety is: living life your way.'

Sam is one of many young women I bond with who are redefining sobriety. There's Bianka Ismailovski — an ethically non-monogamous, pole-dancing, sex-positive comedian and podcaster in her early 30s, who went from self-confessed 'drunken hot mess' to sober queen. She says alcohol got in the way of her really knowing herself, that putting down the bottle has been her greatest act of self-care, and that sobriety continues to be 'the most rewarding, beautiful and joyful experience'.

Then there's Olivia Molly-Rogers, a former Miss Universe Australia, artist, model, and mental health advocate. She joins me on #NoBoozeDayTuesday for a live interview in lockdown in the early days of her sobriety in June 2021, sharing a raw, honest account of how she quit drinking at 29 because it was impacting her mental health and her relationship with her partner.

With a schedule of fashion festivals, socialite parties, and high-end travel, you couldn't find a more glamorous advert for alcohol-free life. Sharing her sobriety with her 180,000 Instagram followers, she's inundated with messages from young women thoroughly sick of their own energy-sapping hangovers and drunken misdeeds, and eager to change.

I'm drawn to these sober women's confidence and how they're reclaiming sobriety as a form of sexy social rebellion. It makes me reflect on how much time I wasted being drunk, and how different my trajectory might have been if I'd had the epiphanies they've had about alcohol at their age. Or when I was a teenager. Instead, I spent my formative years changing myself in a million different ways, trying to erase the parts that felt unacceptable. I chased scraps of approval in an endless bid to belong and to feel like I was enough. Drinking was a big part of that quest for acceptance. It allowed me to reinvent myself. The bookish, quiet girl became the wild child who threw raucous parties when her parents were out of town. I'd pretend to forget that the same girls who had tormented me and told me I was nothing were now toasting me with shots of vodka in my family home. I became Starkers, the party girl, and carried that persona all the way into adulthood. I told myself that being the drunkest person in the room gave me value. But, looking back, I don't see worth in that behaviour. All I see is someone who was drowning. Someone who learned to numb the pain and lost herself along the way.

They say you can't be what you can't see. Women like Sam, Bianka, and Olivia offer a window into a life that was previously hidden from sight. They hold a mirror up for anyone who wants to ditch alcohol but is scared that life will look dull, boring, and friendless without it. When I was binge-drinking in my teens and well into my 30s, there was no representation of sobriety as a fulfilling path. It was always the consolation prize, stigmatised as a lesser life. When I finally did have my first crack at sobriety a decade ago, I felt very much like a lone traveller in a foreign land. Now, I find myself buoyed by this community of sober champions who have put down their wine glasses so they can grab life with both hands.

It feels rebellious to reject the dominant societal script that tells you alcohol is the key to feeling comfortable in your own skin — a script that insists you 'get on the beers' if you want to belong. In a world still obsessed with booze, sobriety is an act of radical defiance. It's an act that says, *I choose me.* There is something deliciously subversive about being part of this burgeoning counterculture. The boring wowsers are becoming the zeitgeist pioneers.

And that's what I want to leave you with. If you're reading this book, I imagine you're questioning your connection with alcohol in some way. Perhaps you've done the online quizzes asking if you're an alcoholic, and perhaps the answer was no, but something still doesn't feel right. Rather than asking whether your drinking is bad enough to quit, ask yourself: Is my life with alcohol in it as good as it could be?

A turning point for me was when I stopped viewing sobriety as deprivation. Instead of fixating on what I was missing, I trained my eye on everything I'd gained: better sleep, reduced anxiety, more energy, improved relationships (with myself and the people I love), greater calm and contentment, and the courage to live my life on my terms. These days, I've swapped FOMO (the fear of missing out) for JOMO (the joy of missing out). I've realised I don't like loud bars and nightclubs and staying out late, and probably never did. I enjoy getting up early and swimming in the ocean; reading a book on the couch under a blanket with my cat curled up next to me; and being home on Saturday night.

I can see that one of the reasons I felt calmer during lockdown was because I was tapping into my true nature. I reconnected with the part of me that values stillness and quiet over the frenetic pace of the life I was living before. The longer I'm sober, the more I understand what I need to sustain me. Now, I take full advantage of one of our greatest untapped resources: Sunday mornings. Rather than mourning the fact that I don't *get* to drink, I celebrate that I don't *have* to drink.

That doesn't mean it's always an easy path. Although things are changing, we still live in a culture where drinking is the dominant social norm, and it can be tiring having to repeatedly explain your choices. And, of course, I still have my battles. But I'm no longer running from them. I've learned that while I sometimes buckle, I never break. There's a steel in my spine that guides me back to my strength when times get tough. I'm not sure I would have found it if I'd continued to use alcohol as an anaesthetic. If the worst thing about sobriety is that you get to feel all your feelings, then the best thing about sobriety is that you get to feel all your feelings. I feel the edges of my pain now, and sometimes they're rough and jagged and they can cut, but I'm also experiencing joy more intensely than I ever have. I get struck by soaring moments of heart-bursting joy —

the kind of pure hedonism I once believed could only be delivered chemically. I can see now that I drank for one of two reasons: to increase pleasure, or to reduce pain. Learning to do both things without alcohol is the definition of true liberation.

I can't categorically state that I'll never drink again. But I don't see a future where alcohol adds anything to my life. Vulnerability researcher Brené Brown says that courage starts with showing up and letting ourselves be seen. Sobriety has allowed me to see myself in dazzling clarity: my frailties and strengths; my petty grievances and deepest desires; the parts I was scared to look at and the parts I didn't know I had. I think that's the greatest gift of all — the capacity to face my own feelings and to realise I'm strong enough to accommodate them.

A friend turned to me at dinner recently, as I sipped my non-alcoholic champagne, and said that in all the years she'd known me, she'd never seen me with such a strong sense of self. This is what sobriety is giving me — the freedom to be who I really am, and to love that person wholeheartedly. It's a reunion with my true self that feels like coming home.

I've excavated the authentic version of me that for so long was buried under the weight of expectation and other people's opinions. Starkers the party girl was a caricature — a performative alter-ego I created as a painfully self-conscious teenager who just wanted to fit in. If I could go back and tell that scared girl anything, it would be that life will get better in ways she can't even imagine when she realises the only approval she needs is her own.

Resources

IF YOU'RE READING this with a head that feels like a bag of sand and a stomach that could churn butter, you'll know by now that I feel your pain. Those drunken adventures can be hilarious, but the hangovers are usually far less fun. If you feel like it's a time for a spell on dry land, there is a rope to help pull you there. Here are some places to start:

Hello Sunday Morning

Since this book first came out, Hello Sunday Morning has grown to an organisation with global reach, and is now a thriving, supportive online community of people who are trying to cut back on drinking, taking a break from alcohol, or have quit altogether.

Their Daybreak app takes an evidence-based approach to reducing alcohol consumption, using health coaches and peer-to-peer support to help keep you on track.

hellosundaymorning.org

This Naked Mind

Annie Grace's This Naked Mind is a book, a podcast, and an online movement that empowers you to take gain control of your drinking. It has range of really helpful free resources, including The Alcohol

Experiment, a 30-day action plan that can help change the way you think about the role of alcohol in your life.

thisnakedmind.com

Tempest

Founded by *Quit Like a Woman* author Holly Whitaker, Tempest is a membership-based recovery program with clinically proven tools that takes a holistic approach to understanding why you drink and what strategies you need to quit.

jointempest.com

Sober Mates

An online community founded by Sam Wilson that serves as an educational platform to explore your drinking habits and to shake up drinking expectations. It's a judgement-free space full of inspiration and motivation, and you don't need to be sober to be part of it.

Sam regularly hosts in-person events in Australia and a regular sober book club online.

sobermates.com.au

Sober Girl Society

Millie Gooch started Sober Girl Society as an Instagram page, which has turned into a movement with followers all over the world. She describes it as a 'sisterly safe space for sober and sober curious women who are changing their relationship with alcohol'.

Millie also hosts real-life meetups in the UK for sober socialising, and is the author of *The Sober Girl Society Handbook*.

sobergirlsociety.com

Clinical support

If you need more support to quit drinking, it's always a good idea to talk to a GP first, particularly if you feel you may be physically dependent. They will be able to give you advice tailor-made to your circumstances, and refer you for further treatment if necessary.

Acknowledgements

WHEN I WAS writing this book, I had an outstanding support crew. True friends are those who see you at your worst — during the tears, tantrums, and trips down the rabbit hole — and love you anyway. For that, I thank you, Nat, Mel, and Bach; and I also thank you for your endless patience and advice, and for those days at work when you put me back together and reminded me to keep breathing.

Likewise, Amy, my rock, thanks for those long telephone conversations well into the night. When I was so confused that I couldn't see straight, you made the path ahead clear.

Lisa, my oldest friend, and one of the most incredible women I know, thank you so much. Without your help, the hardest parts of this book might never have been written.

Similarly, Mari-Claire, your open heart and willingness to listen saved me from being pulled under when things were bleak. I'll never forget it.

Ben, my very first proofreader — I'm so grateful for your generosity, honesty, and PR disaster-planning. Your kind words sustained me and gave me faith that I was on the right track.

And kudos to you, Timmy, the pillar that props up our inner-north crew, for not questioning why a journalist/would-be-author didn't have her own printer when I asked to print a 300-page manuscript on yours, 12 hours before deadline.

Chris Raine, who navigated this year-long boozeless odyssey before me, and talked me down from the ledge when those bottles of wine became too tempting, thanks for letting me be part of the extraordinary movement you started.

At Scribe, thanks to Henry Rosenbloom and Julia Carlomagno for taking a punt on this binge-drinking health reporter. Your judicious and gentle editing made the process far less painful than I'd anticipated. Thanks also to Allison Colpoys and Miriam Rosenbloom for the kick-arse cover art, to Ian See for the diligent proofreading, and to Cora Roberts for being the best publicist in the business.

To my former *Sunday Age* editor Gay Alcorn, thanks for your support and patience as I took time off to finish this book. I'm a better writer for having you as a mentor. Thanks also to your successor, Mark Forbes, for being so accommodating about my book commitments.

I'm incredibly grateful to all the people in the alcohol and drug sector who have helped me, not only with this book, but also throughout my six years of covering alcohol issues for *The Age* and *The Sunday Age*. But I'd particularly like to thank Jon Currie, Rob Moodie, John Rogerson, and Geoff Munro, who have gone out of their way to assist me from day one. Special mention to Renee Lustman, too, for assisting with my research, and for never being flummoxed by my many requests, no matter how obscure.

To my friends Nick, Cat, Tony, and Brigitte, thanks for sharing your experiences with (and without) alcohol. Your generosity made my job easy. Likewise, to all the people in Australia and Scotland who I interviewed — colleagues, fellow *HSM*-ers, academics, specialists, and strangers — I can't thank you enough for your insights into our drinking culture. You told your stories with lived knowledge, honesty, and bravery. This is as much your book as mine.

Above all, I'm indebted to the two women who grounded me, nurtured me, put up with my erratic moods, and made sure that I ate and left the house during that long summer of writing — my soul sisters, Loretta and Kath. Thank you doesn't even come close. Your friendship is my anchor.

To the many wonderful friends who have come into my life since the first edition of this book was published, I thank you for your love and support. Special shout out to the vibrant women I've met in the sober space, who make sobriety hellasexy. And particular thanks to Nonie, Jason, Chris, Tash, Rania, Sarah, Ben, Tammy, Nick, Lallo, and Cass, my Melbourne family who have kept me afloat when the water was choppy. I love you all.

And I couldn't have written this book without the support of my incredible family. Neil, Ker, Daisy, and Orla — my personal cheer squad — your encouragement gives me the belief that I can do anything. Dad, thank you for the writing genes you passed on, and for your unwavering faith in me throughout my life. Your love and support have helped me more than you'll ever know. Mum, you taught me the importance of living life as if no-one's watching. Thank you (and sorry) for all those late-night, incoherent phone calls, for dancing with me on bar tops and in steam trains, and for loving me with a ferocity that makes the miles irrelevant.

Finally, to Fiona, the girl I have loved my whole life — heartfelt thanks for a friendship that continues to nourish and inspire me, and most of all for letting me share Jude's life with the world. Your sparkly little boy has changed everything.